COMPACT *Research*

Brain Tumors

Diseases and Disorders

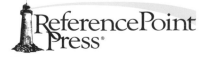

ReferencePoint
Press®

San Diego, CA

Select* books in the Compact Research series include:

Current Issues

Animal Experimentation
Conflict in the Middle East
Disaster Response
DNA Evidence and
    Investigation
Drugs and Sports
Gangs
Genetic Testing
Gun Control
Immigration
Islam
National Security
Nuclear Weapons and
    Security
Obesity
Religious Fundamentalism
Stem Cells
Teen Smoking
Terrorist Attacks
Video Games

Diseases and Disorders

ADHD
Anxiety Disorders
Bipolar Disorders
Drug Addiction
Herpes
HPV
Influenza
Mood Disorders
Obsessive-Compulsive
    Disorder
Personality Disorders
Post-Traumatic Stress
    Disorder
Self-Injury Disorder
Sexually Transmitted
    Diseases

Drugs

Antidepressants
Club Drugs
Cocaine and Crack
Hallucinogens
Heroin
Inhalants
Methamphetamine
Nicotine and Tobacco
Painkillers
Performance-Enhancing
    Drugs
Prescription Drugs
Steroids

Energy and the Environment

Biofuels
Coal Power
Deforestation
Energy Alternatives
Garbage and Recycling
Global Warming and
    Climate Change
Hydrogen Power
Nuclear Power
Oil Spills and Offshore
    Drilling
Solar Power
Toxic Waste
Wind Power

*For a complete list of titles please visit www.referencepointpress.com.

Brain Tumors

Peggy J. Parks

Diseases and Disorders

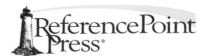

ReferencePoint
Press®

San Diego, CA

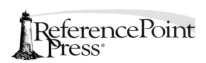

© 2011 ReferencePoint Press, Inc.
Printed in the United States

For more information, contact:
ReferencePoint Press, Inc.
PO Box 27779
San Diego, CA 92198
www.ReferencePointPress.com

Picture credits:
Cover: Dreamstime and iStockphoto.com
Maury Aaseng: 32–34, 46–48, 60–62, 74–76
© Corbis: 12
Scott Camazine/Science Photo Library: 19

LIBRARY OF CONGRESS CATALOGING-IN-PUBLICATION DATA

Parks, Peggy J., 1951–
    Brain tumors / By Peggy J. Parks.
        p. cm. — (Compact research)
    Includes bibliographical references and index.
    ISBN-13: 978-1-60152-138-5 (hardcover)
    ISBN-10: 1-60152-138-3 (hardcover)
    1. Brain—Tumors—Popular works. I. Title.
    RC280.B7P37   2011
    616.99'481—dc22
                                                        2010040107

Contents

Foreword

❝Where is the knowledge we have lost in information?❞

—T.S. Eliot, "The Rock."

As modern civilization continues to evolve, its ability to create, store, distribute, and access information expands exponentially. The explosion of information from all media continues to increase at a phenomenal rate. By 2020 some experts predict the worldwide information base will double every 73 days. While access to diverse sources of information and perspectives is paramount to any democratic society, information alone cannot help people gain knowledge and understanding. Information must be organized and presented clearly and succinctly in order to be understood. The challenge in the digital age becomes not the creation of information, but how best to sort, organize, enhance, and present information.

ReferencePoint Press developed the *Compact Research* series with this challenge of the information age in mind. More than any other subject area today, researching current issues can yield vast, diverse, and unqualified information that can be intimidating and overwhelming for even the most advanced and motivated researcher. The *Compact Research* series offers a compact, relevant, intelligent, and conveniently organized collection of information covering a variety of current topics ranging from illegal immigration and deforestation to diseases such as anorexia and meningitis.

The series focuses on three types of information: objective single-author narratives, opinion-based primary source quotations, and facts and statistics. The clearly written objective narratives provide context and reliable background information. Primary source quotes are carefully selected and cited, exposing the reader to differing points of view. And facts and statistics sections aid the reader in evaluating perspectives. Presenting these key types of information creates a richer, more balanced learning experience.

For better understanding and convenience, the series enhances information by organizing it into narrower topics and adding design features that make it easy for a reader to identify desired content. For example, in *Compact Research: Illegal Immigration*, a chapter covering the economic impact of illegal immigration has an objective narrative explaining the various ways the economy is impacted, a balanced section of numerous primary source quotes on the topic, followed by facts and full-color illustrations to encourage evaluation of contrasting perspectives.

The ancient Roman philosopher Lucius Annaeus Seneca wrote, "It is quality rather than quantity that matters." More than just a collection of content, the *Compact Research* series is simply committed to creating, finding, organizing, and presenting the most relevant and appropriate amount of information on a current topic in a user-friendly style that invites, intrigues, and fosters understanding.

Brain Tumors at a Glance

How Brain Tumors Form

Brain tumors form when cells begin growing out of control and coagulate into a mass of abnormal tissue.

Primary and Secondary Tumors

Tumors that originate in the brain are known as primary brain tumors, while secondary tumors form when cancers in other parts of the body spread to the brain.

Grades of Brain Tumors

Brain tumors are classified according to how their cells appear under a microscope, as well as their severity, and are assigned grades from 1 to 4.

Prevalence

The Brain Science Foundation estimates that 612,000 people in the United States are living with a primary brain tumor.

Symptoms

People with brain tumors may have a sudden onset of headaches, as well as suffer from seizures, nausea, vision problems, and/or hearing loss.

Causes

Scientists do not know what causes primary brain tumors but theorize that genetic mutations, exposure to radiation, and other environmental factors may play a role.

Risks of Brain Tumors

Brain tumors can take up space within the skull and damage healthy tissue, as well as affect eyesight, hearing, and movement. People with some cancerous tumors have a high risk of death.

Effectiveness of Treatment

Technology such as magnetic resonance imaging, improved surgical techniques, and other sophisticated treatment methods have vastly improved people's chances of surviving a brain tumor.

Overview

In early 2009, when fashion designer and actress Tara Subkoff began to suffer from blinding headaches, she knew something was wrong. Her doctor was convinced that it was nothing more than TMJ, the same jaw disorder that her mother had. But then Subkoff's headaches got even more painful, she started having bouts of dizziness, and was losing her hearing in one ear. "I remember thinking that diagnosis didn't sound quite right," she says. "It felt like something was different, like it was worse."[1] Her suspicion was confirmed when a magnetic resonance imaging (MRI) scan showed a golf ball–sized tumor on the right side of her brain.

On September 10, 2009, Subkoff underwent a 14-hour operation, during which surgeons were able to remove the entire tumor. To her immense relief, pathology tests indicated that the tumor was benign rather than cancerous. She made it through the surgery just fine, but she endured many difficult months during her recovery and suffered some lasting ef-fects. For instance, she lost full hear-ing in her right ear and developed vertigo, which is a constant sensa-tion of spinning or whirling caused by damage to nerves that control balance. Also, for the rest of her life, Subkoff will have to undergo regular MRIs. Even though benign tumors do not usually grow back, regrowth is a possibility, so doctors want to monitor her brain to ensure that the tumor does not return.

> " **Primary brain tumors may be benign and slow growing, or ma-lignant, meaning they are composed of cancer cells and grow rapidly.** "

In spite of all she has gone through, Subkoff feels extremely fortunate and says that the frightening experience has given her a new outlook on life. "So much of this time has been about appreciating life in the moment," she writes. "If you focus, you will discover that even the hard ones have something beautiful to them. Life is so fast, it feels important to stop and freeze and appreciate the now."[2]

What Are Brain Tumors?

For an organ that weighs only about 3 pounds (1.4kg), the brain holds an inconceivable amount of power. It controls everything people do, from thinking and learning to imagining, dreaming, and remembering. The brain also regulates body movement, making it possible to sip a cup of coffee, dribble a ball down a basketball court, send a text message, or even scratch an itch. As neurosurgeon Keith Black writes: "Unlike any other organ in the body, our brain is the essence of what makes us hu-man, our memories, our thoughts, our personalities—one hundred bil-lion nerve cells, working in absolute harmony to allow us to see, to smell, to move, to understand, and to create."[3]

Black's reference to cells is important because brain tumors originate in cells. All the cells in the body, including those that make up the brain, are kept in check through a process known as apoptosis. When cells grow

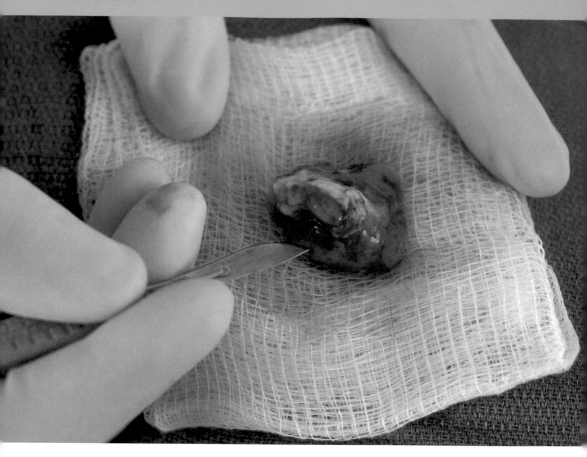

Biopsy, or the surgical removal of a tissue sample from a tumor, is standard procedure for most patients with a brain tumor. A tumor removed for biopsy, such as the one shown here, helps doctors confirm their diagnosis and determine the tumor's grade and speed of growth.

old, become damaged, or are exposed to some type of infection, they die a natural death. As this is happening, new cells are being generated to replace those that have died. But sometimes, for reasons that are not well understood, the process goes awry. Old or damaged cells do not die as they should, and new cells start forming and multiplying when the body does not need them. If cells continue to grow, divide, and produce more cells, they can coagulate into a mass of abnormal tissue known as a tumor.

When this sort of mass develops in the brain, it is known as a primary brain tumor. The term is used to refer to tumors that originate in the central nervous system, which includes the brain, spinal cord, and meninges, the layers of tissue that protect the brain and spinal cord. Primary brain tumors may be benign and slow growing, or malignant, meaning they are composed of cancer cells and grow rapidly.

Unlike primary brain tumors, secondary tumors do not originate in the brain. Rather, they begin as cancer in other parts of the body. In a process known as metastasis, cancerous cells break off from the main cancer site and travel through the bloodstream to the central nervous system. Once they have established themselves, the cells begin to grow and multiply rapidly, forming one or more secondary (metastatic) brain tumors.

Tiny Cells, Gigantic Jobs

Because brain tumors arise from cells, knowing what these cells are and the roles they play in brain function helps to better understand tumors. Neurons are like the chips of a supercomputer, highly specialized cells that continuously send messages to and from each other in the form of electrochemical signals. As the authors of the book *Your Brain After Chemo* explain: "Every time we balance our checkbooks or look for our keys or realize we forgot to defrost the chicken—every sensory experience, every emotion and mood, every voluntary move of our bodies, every single thought that occurs to us—all correspond to some neurons firing off messages to many others."[4]

As essential as neurons are for brain functioning, they could not perform their work without the assistance of glial cells, or glia. Their importance was unknown for many years, with scientists focusing their attention solely on neurons. A Stanford School of Medicine article explains: "Glial cells' activities are subtler than those of neurons—unlike their flashier electronic cousins, they converse in biochemical whispers."[5] Glial cells provide nourishment and physical support to neurons, as well as protect them against foreign invaders such as bacteria and viruses. And glia are

> " One important difference between malignant tumors in the brain and those in other parts of the body is that brain tumors almost never spread to other organs. "

far more plentiful than neurons, comprising nearly 90 percent of the brain's cells.

Glia are divided into subtypes, with each playing its own supportive role to neurons. Oligodendrocytes, for example, insulate neurons by wrapping their axons (long wire-like tails) in a protective sheath known as myelin. This is a crucial function, as the University of Utah Genetic Science Learning Center explains: "The job of these cells is to speed up the electrical signal (action potential) that travels down an axon. Without oligodendrocytes an action potential would travel down an axon 30 times slower!"[6]

Astrocytes, the most abundant of all glia, are so named because they appear star shaped under a microscope (*astro* is the Greek word for "star"). Astrocytes hold neurons in place, furnish them with nutrients, and digest parts of dead neurons. Microglia are special immune cells that are found only in the brain. They have the ability to detect damaged or unhealthy neurons and protect neurons by eating bacteria and viruses. Two other types of glia are Schwann cells, which wrap around nerve fibers to help support and insulate them; and satellite cells, which provide physical support to neurons throughout the central nervous system.

> "Children may also suffer from seizures, although only a small number of childhood seizures are caused by brain tumors."

Brain Tumor Categories

Primary brain tumors are often named after the types of cells that comprise them. Although primary tumors can develop from neurons, as well as from meninges and other tissue, they usually develop from glial cells to form tumors known as gliomas. The most common type of glioma is the astrocytoma, which arises from astrocytes.

Brain tumors are classified according to their severity and appearance, with each assigned a grade from 1 to 4 (often called low grade or high grade). One of the criteria is how tumor cells look when they are viewed under a microscope. For instance, normal cells tend to have a consistent size and shape, while cancerous cells have an abnormal appearance with varying sizes and shapes. The American Cancer Society explains: "They may be either smaller or larger than normal cells. Normal cells often have certain shapes that help them better do their jobs. Cancer cells usually do not function in a useful way and their shapes are often distorted."[7]

The benign and slow-growing grade 1 glioma looks almost normal under a microscope. Grade 2 gliomas, which are malignant but relatively slow growing, are composed of cells that have a slightly abnormal appearance. The cancerous cells that make up grade 3 gliomas are actively reproducing, and when viewed under a microscope, they look quite abnormal. The most malignant, aggressive, and dangerous brain tumors are those in the grade 4 category. These have the most abnormal appearance of all tumors, are composed of rapidly multiplying cancerous cells, and are able to perpetuate their own growth by forming new blood vessels.

> " People with grade 4 brain tumors have a high risk of death because the cancer spreads rapidly, invading and destroying brain tissue. "

One important difference between malignant tumors in the brain and those in other parts of the body is that brain tumors almost never spread to other organs. Although they do metastasize, their spread tends to remain confined to the central nervous system. Don M. Long, who is a professor in the neurology department at Johns Hopkins Hospital, explains: "Some cancers of other organs are called malignant because they cause death by spreading throughout the body. Brain tumors rarely spread in this way. For brain tumors, the word malignant means they cause death because they grow (or grow back) rapidly in the same place where they originate, not because they affect other organs."[8]

Who Suffers from Brain Tumors?

Brain tumors can strike anyone, from newborn babies to octogenarians. According to the Brain Science Foundation, more than 612,000 people in the United States are currently living with a primary tumor of the brain or spinal cord. Brain tumors affect both males and females, as well as people of all races and walks of life. Some populations do, however, have a slightly higher risk than others. In general, primary brain tumors affect males more often than females, although a few types are more prominent among women. Studies have also shown that non-Hispanic Caucasians are more likely to develop primary brain tumors than African Americans or Hispanics.

The prevalence of secondary brain tumors is more challenging for health officials to gauge, but they do compile approximate figures. The American Brain Tumor Association writes: "Although statistics for brain metastases are not readily available, it is estimated that more than 150,000 cancer patients per year will have symptoms due to a metastatic brain tumor or a metastatic brain tumor in the spinal cord."[9] The group adds that secondary brain tumors are at least four times as common in adults as primary brain tumors.

The reverse is true in children and adolescents, in whom primary brain tumors are far more common. Primary brain tumors represent the second most frequent malignancy among children, second only to leukemia (cancer of the blood or bone marrow) as the leading cause of childhood cancer-related deaths. The Pediatric Brain Tumor Foundation reports that in the United States, 28,000 children and youth aged 19 and under are living with the diagnosis of a primary brain tumor, with more than three-fourths younger than 15.

Warning Signs

Different parts of the brain control different mental and physical functions, so brain tumor symptoms vary depending on where the tumor is located. In the earliest stages of a brain tumor, there may be no symptoms at all. As the tumor begins to grow, headaches may develop, which gradually become more frequent and severe over time. Other symptoms include vomiting, with or without nausea; problems with eyesight such as blurred vision, double vision, or loss of peripheral vision; and hearing loss. People may experience a gradual loss of sensation and/or movement in an arm or a leg, or a loss of balance. They may have problems thinking, speaking, or finding the right words to express their thoughts, and may become easily confused and disoriented.

Seizures are also common in people with brain tumors. According to the American Brain Tumor Association, up to 40 percent of brain tumor patients have a seizure at some time during their illness. These may be tonic clonic (grand mal) seizures, during which the person experiences violent, convulsive movements and loses consciousness. Or seizures may be milder, evoking strange feelings and sensations such as seeing, smelling, and hearing things that are not actually there.

Children may also suffer from seizures, although only a small number of childhood seizures are caused by brain tumors. Many common brain tumor symptoms are not noticeable in children because they may be mistaken for those of normal childhood illnesses. Neurosurgeon Peter M. Black writes: "Slow-growing tumors may cause symptoms to appear gradually, so children and their parents do not initially connect headaches, school difficulties, or clumsiness with a growth in the brain. Pediatricians may also suspect that particular symptoms are caused by sinus infections, intestinal problems, viruses, or other illnesses much more common in childhood than cancer."[10]

What Causes Brain Tumors?

Although it is known that primary brain tumors arise from a buildup of abnormal cells, why this happens is largely a mystery. In children, research suggests that genetic mutations (errors in genes) play a role in disrupting apoptosis, which could lead to the uncontrolled cell growth that causes tumors to develop. Children's Hospital Boston explains:

> There are many ways to damage a cell's control. Most pediatric brain tumors are thought to arise from an accident during normal cellular division that creates a mutant gene. A mutated gene may tell a cell to continue dividing; like having your foot stuck on the gas pedal, or it may not tell a cell to stop; like having no brakes. Either way, the cells divide in a way that they shouldn't, creating a tumor.[11]

In addition to genetic mutations, several environmental risk factors for primary brain tumors have been identified. One is exposure to ionized radiation, the high-dose X-ray therapy that is used to treat cancer. According to the National Institutes of Health, radiation therapy to the head, which is used to treat brain cancers, increases the risk for brain tumors up to 20 or 30 years afterward.

In many adults, however, there is no plausible reason why primary brain tumors develop. The tumors cannot be explained by genetics, and exposure to radiation is not a factor. As Marc Chamberlain, a neurology professor and director of the Brain Tumor Program at the University of Washington, explains: "We don't know what causes them. For all practical purposes, they tend to come out of nowhere."[12]

The cause of secondary brain tumors is more clear-cut because they metastasize from cancers elsewhere in the body. Many types of cancer can spread to the brain, but some have been shown to do so more often than others. For instance, people with breast, lung, kidney, or colon cancer have a particularly high risk of developing metastatic brain tumors. One of the most common types of cancer to spread to the brain is melanoma, which is a malignancy of pigment-producing cells known as melanocytes. These cells are located primarily in the skin, but are also found in the eyes, ears, gastrointestinal tract, and oral and genital mucous membranes.

What Are the Risks of Brain Tumors?

The degree of risk or danger to a patient can vary widely depending on the type, size, and location of the tumor. The National Brain Tumor Society explains: "The growth of a tumor takes up space within the skull and interferes with normal brain activity. A tumor can cause damage by increasing pressure in the brain, by shifting the brain or pushing against the skull, and by invading and damaging nerves and healthy brain tissue."[13] Benign brain tumors can be as dangerous as malignant tumors if they are located in a vital area, such as the brain stem or spinal cord.

People with grade 4 brain tumors have a high risk of death because the cancer spreads rapidly, invading and destroying brain tissue. This is the case with the glioblastoma multiforme, which is among the deadliest tumors. Keith Black is intimately familiar with the tumor because he has seen it ravage the brains of far too many patients. He refers to it as "an enemy I have known for a long time, and one that I no doubt will be battling for years to come. This tumor spreads through the brain like a wildfire, consuming critical brain tissue in its path. . . . A glioblastoma can double in size in fourteen days."[14] Senator Edward Kennedy was diagnosed with a glioblastoma in May 2008 and underwent surgery, followed by radiation and chemotherapy treatments. The tumor continued to spread, however, and Kennedy died 15 months later at the age of 77.

Diagnosis and Treatment

If a patient exhibits symptoms that could possibly indicate a brain tumor, a physician will usually recommend a neurological workup. This includes an examination of vision, hearing, balance, coordination, and reflexes. Imaging tests, such as an MRI, a computerized tomography scan, and/or a positron-emission tomography scan, are commonly performed if a brain tumor is suspected. If one or more of these imaging tests indicates the presence of a tumor, a neurologist will determine the best way to proceed and make a recommendation to the patient and his or her family.

The treatment that is recommended for a brain tumor differs based on the type, grade, and size of the tumor, as well as its location in the

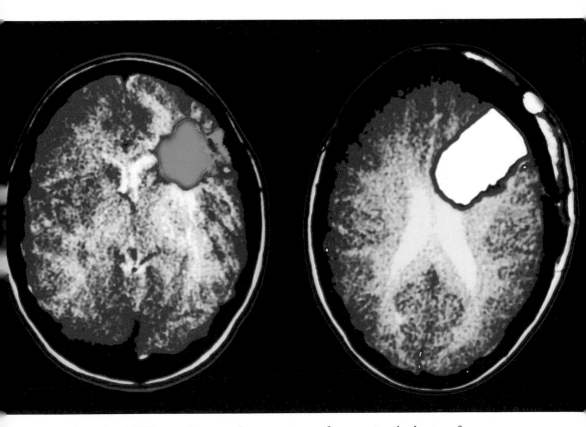

A cerebral CT scan shows a glioma, a type of tumor, in the brain of a 16-year-old girl before and after surgery. The tumor (shown in green) is visible in the image on the left. The image on the right shows where the tumor and surrounding tissue were removed. Eighty percent of malignant tumors are gliomas.

> " Although brain tumors can pose serious health risks, sophisticated treatment methods are enabling many people to survive longer than ever before. This is true not only of benign tumors, but of malignant tumors as well. "

central nervous system. Once a tumor has been diagnosed, treatment decisions may need to be made quickly, especially if it is determined that the tumor is operable. Many types of tumors grow unbelievably fast, and even a few hours can make a difference in a patient's survival and long-term health.

Following surgery to remove a brain tumor, radiation therapy will likely be used as a supplemental treatment. This is true for many types of tumors, including all grades. Lisa M. DeAngelis, who is chair of the Department of Neurology at the Memorial Sloan-Kettering Cancer Center, explains: "Even low-grade gliomas cannot be cured by surgery alone because individual cells migrate great distances within the brain tissue, and a surgeon cannot remove large portions of the brain without causing unacceptable damage. Depending on the type of tumor, therefore, oncologists may recommend radiation after surgery."[15]

How Successful Are Brain Tumor Treatments?

Although brain tumors can pose serious health risks, sophisticated treatment methods are enabling many people to survive longer than ever before. This is true not only of benign tumors, but of malignant tumors as well. According to 2009 data by the National Cancer Institute, 23.7 percent of people diagnosed in 1977 with brain cancer survived for 5 years. By 2006 the 5-year survival rate had increased to more than 36 percent. As medical science continues to reveal more about brain tumors and new treatments are developed, the survival rate will undoubtedly continue to improve—and perhaps someday scientists will find a cure for this potentially deadly medical condition.

What Are Brain Tumors?

> **'Tumor' is a general term describing new growth of cells in an inappropriate manner (i.e. serving no useful purpose).**
>
> —Brain Science Foundation, which seeks to increase awareness of primary brain tumors and to make brain tumor research a priority.

> **A diagnosis of a brain tumor can be overwhelming and frightening. It can make you feel like you have little control over your health.**
>
> —Mayo Clinic, a world-renowned medical facility that is headquartered in Rochester, Minnesota.

Most people would not consider it a blessing to be involved in a bus accident. But for Caitlin DeVoll, a 16-year-old girl from the small Michigan town of Copemish, that is exactly what it was. A cheerleader and member of her high school track team, DeVoll had suffered from headaches, dizziness, memory loss, vision problems, and fatigue for five years. The symptoms began when she was 11, soon after she had fallen off a swing and landed on her head. She was taken to a hospital in nearby Traverse City, where doctors performed an MRI and diagnosed a mild concussion. They could see a small spot on the MRI scan but determined that it was cerebrospinal fluid, a clear fluid that surrounds the brain and spinal cord. That conclusion, however, later proved to be flawed.

The Correct Diagnosis

The bus accident happened on March 12, 2010. DeVoll was riding in a school bus when another vehicle struck it, and the impact threw her into a window, causing her to hit the left side of her head. Two days later she was having such severe headaches that she was taken to a larger hospital 125 miles (201km) away in Grand Rapids. She underwent an MRI, and a specialist finally discovered what her problem had been all along—a brain tumor. By comparing the MRI from 2005 with the new scan, the doctor could see how the tumor in DeVoll's brain had grown. The spot that was visible on the older scan looked like a tiny bubble, and over 5 years it had developed into a tumor that measured nearly 1 inch (2.5cm) across. The neurosurgeon showed the scans to DeVoll's mother and said: "That's what everybody's been missing."[16]

> " Tumors can form anywhere in the body, including the brain, and the one trait they share in common is that they all develop from cells. "

DeVoll underwent two brain operations, and pathology tests showed that the tumor was malignant. Surgeons were able to get most of it out, but not all, because part of the tumor was intertwined with a ventricle, one of the cavities in the brain that produce, store, and drain cerebrospinal fluid. A small piece could not be removed without risking serious brain damage. She will need to undergo MRIs every three to four months so doctors can monitor the tumor fragment and make sure it does not grow.

DeVoll's life has changed since she learned that she has brain cancer. She is again involved with band, but cannot participate in cheerleading or track because of the risk that she might hit her head, which could possibly jar the tumor into regrowth. Yet in spite of all that she has gone through, and the uncertainties that undoubtedly lie ahead, she has an amazing spirit and a renewed zest for life. "I live one day at a time," she says. "I don't take life for granted—every day is a gift."[17]

Cells and Tumor Growth

The word *tumor* is often assumed to be a synonym for *cancer*, but that is not necessarily correct. Although the very idea of having a tumor may be frightening, tumors are not always cancerous; in fact, the majority are benign. They can form anywhere in the body, including the brain, and the one trait they share in common is that they all develop from cells.

Most of the body's cells lie on a thin, net-like mesh known as the extracellular matrix, which is composed of proteins. Donald Ingber, who is a senior associate in pathology and surgery at Children's Hospital Boston, says that the extracellular matrix "not only gives the cells something to connect to, it also helps to tell each cell which way is up and where it is in relation to its neighbors." This protein mesh supports cells and maintains the structure and form of the body's tissue, as Ingber explains: "Cells die off and are replaced many times during our lifetimes, but the mesh acts like a physical memory. It is what keeps us looking like us throughout our lives."[18]

The extracellular matrix plays a pivotal role in the cell changes that lead to tumor formation. Even though apoptosis is a tightly controlled process, cells sometimes start dividing even though there is no room for them to spread. Ingber writes: "With no space on the underlying mesh, the new cells begin to pile up. Because they are not in contact with the mesh, they don't orient themselves correctly, and so normal tissue structure and function are lost. If the cells continue to divide, the cell structure becomes a random pile of disoriented cells. In other words, it's a tumor." At this point, the "pile" of cells is still above the underlying protein mesh, so the tumor may disappear on its own. Ingber explains: "Because normal cells need to touch the mesh to survive, the piled-up cells die away and normal tissue form is restored."[19]

> " Most people who develop malignant brain tumors have cancer elsewhere in their bodies that has spread to the brain. "

In some cases, however, the abnormal cells do not die, and the tumor keeps growing. For unknown reasons, the piled-up cells are able to survive and grow without touching the extracellular matrix. In the brain this results in a primary tumor, which is benign as long as its cells remain above the protein mesh. But sometimes cells develop the ability to break through the mesh, invade neighboring tissue, and pass through blood vessels. Ingber writes: "These tumors have become 'malignant' or what is commonly known as cancers."[20]

When Cancer Travels to the Brain

Most people who develop malignant brain tumors have cancer elsewhere in their bodies that has spread to the brain. This is known as a secondary brain tumor, but is more commonly referred to as metastatic brain cancer or brain metastases. The cancer that has spread is known as the primary cancer (not to be confused with primary brain tumor). The University of California–San Francisco Medical Center explains: "Cancer that spreads to the brain is the same disease and has the same name as the original or primary cancer. For example, if lung cancer spreads to the brain, the disease is called metastatic lung cancer because the cells in the secondary tumor resemble abnormal lung cells, not abnormal brain cells."[21]

One man whose cancer spread to his brain is Scott Erdman. In the 1980s he was diagnosed with melanoma and underwent several surgeries to remove malignant tumors. Then in 1991, after he started having severe headaches, Erdman underwent an MRI that revealed three metastatic tumors in his brain, one of which was the size of an orange. At the time, he had no sign of melanoma elsewhere in his body, so Keith Black was confident that brain surgery could save the man's life. Black writes: "When a metastatic tumor comes to the brain, it's critical to know how well the disease is controlled elsewhere. If the disease is all over the body, there's no point in treating the brain tumor."[22] Erdman developed another brain tumor the following year and had it removed. Since then, Black says Erdman has remained cancer free.

> A common perception about tumors is that if they are benign, they are harmless—but that is erroneous.

In many cases by the time a secondary brain tumor is discovered, the person's cancer has widely metastasized. Thus, as Black explains, the brain tumor may be an indication that the cancer is out of control. But on occasion, a secondary brain tumor is found before the patient's primary cancer has been discovered. This is known as a metastasis of unknown origin, as the Memorial Sloan-Kettering Cancer Center explains: "These tumors can develop when a patient's primary cancer, while still undetectable at its original site, sends out metastatic cells that travel to the brain and establish themselves there. In these patients, physicians can sometimes biopsy the tumor (depending on its location in the brain), identify the type of cells it is composed of, and determine its site of origin."[23]

A Misleading Term

A common perception about tumors is that if they are benign, they are harmless—but that is erroneous. Benign tumors do not metastasize, as they are not composed of malignant cells that can break away from the cancer site and infiltrate neighboring tissue, but they can grow and spread and wreak havoc on the brain. Cancer specialist Christopher Dolinsky explains:

> One of the special characteristics of brain tumors is that benign (non-cancerous) tumors . . . can be just as bad as malignant (cancerous) brain tumors. This is because the brain is such an important organ. It is locked into place by the skull and can't move out of the way if a tumor is growing near it. Even a benign tumor can cause pressure on the brain, and this pressure can be both symptomatic and life-threatening.[24]

Olivia Briggs, a college student from Keller, Texas, was diagnosed with a benign tumor on her brain stem when she was 11 years old. On more than one occasion, people have told her how lucky she is that her tumor was benign, rather than malignant. She writes: "Normally, you'd be jumping up and down and going crazy inside with excitement that, although [you] have something inside your brain that obviously is not supposed to be there, it's not 'technically' hurting you because the cells composing this tumor are normal and thus noncancerous."[25] From her own personal experience, however, Briggs knows that the word *benign* can be deceptive. Since her tumor is on the brain stem, surgery would be too risky. Her doctors are doing what she calls "watching and waiting," giving

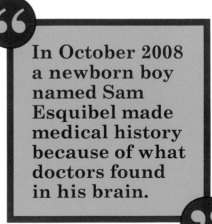

In October 2008 a newborn boy named Sam Esquibel made medical history because of what doctors found in his brain.

her regular MRIs so they can monitor the tumor's growth.

Living with constant uncertainty is stressful for Briggs. She knows that if the tumor grows bigger, it could squeeze her brain stem and cause serious problems with brain function, as well as interfere with breathing and heart rate, which could be life threatening. She is also aware that benign brain tumors can become malignant over time. All she can do is wait—and hope.

A Bizarre Discovery

Brain tumors in little children are uncommon, and are even rarer in babies. But in October 2008 a newborn boy named Sam Esquibel made medical history because of what doctors found in his brain. An ultrasound that was done before Sam's birth showed that he had a large brain tumor, and two days after he was born, neurosurgeon Paul Grabb performed an operation to remove it. Grabb made an incision in Sam's skull—and was totally shocked when a tiny foot slid out. He explains: "A lot of us who have been in practice long enough like to think we've seen everything. Well, we haven't. The foot quite literally popped out of the tumor. I stopped operating, since I'm not used to seeing a foot in the brain."[26] After taking a short break Grabb finished removing the tumor, and found that it also contained pieces of intestine, as well as a partially formed second foot, hand, and thigh.

The pathology report identified the mass as a teratoma, a tumor that forms in a developing fetus and is composed of tissue such as skin and muscle, and/or bits of bone, teeth, and hair. The possibility exists, however, that it was not a teratoma, but rather a fetus in fetu, a rare developmental abnormality in which a fetus forms inside of its twin. According to Grabb, there is a very fine line between the two. But whatever Sam's tumor was, Grabb says nothing he has observed in his career as a surgeon has ever compared to it. He explains: "You show those pictures to the most experienced pediatric neurosurgeons in the world, and they've never seen anything like it."[27]

A Complex Medical Issue

Brain tumors are puzzling and unpredictable, even to physicians who see them every day. It is mysterious that cells somehow begin to grow uncontrollably, pile up, and form the lump of tissue known as a brain tumor, which may be benign or malignant. For people who have cancer elsewhere in their bodies, cells may break away from the primary cancer site, migrate toward the brain, and lodge there, where they rapidly grow and divide to form a metastatic brain tumor. Through years of research, scientists have learned a great deal about brain tumors—but they are the first to say that a great deal remains unknown.

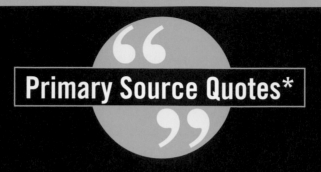

Primary Source Quotes*

What Are Brain Tumors?

"There are a great many different types of brain tumors, each with its own specific biology and treatment, but all cause similar symptoms."

—Lisa M. DeAngelis, "Brain Tumors—The Dana Guide," Dana Foundation, *The Dana Guide to Brain Health*, June 2009. www.dana.org.

DeAngelis is chair of the Department of Neurology at the Memorial Sloan-Kettering Cancer Center.

....

"Brain tumors afflict people of any age—from tiny babies to older persons—with equal ferocity, regardless of background, race, or geographic location."

—Denis Strangman and Kathy Oliver, foreword to *100 Questions & Answers About Brain Tumors*, by Virginia Stark-Vance and M.L. Dubay. Sudbury, MA: Jones and Bartlett, 2011.

Strangman is chair of the International Brain Tumor Alliance, and Oliver is the organization's codirector.

....

* Editor's Note: While the definition of a primary source can be narrowly or broadly defined, for the purposes of Compact Research, a primary source consists of: 1) results of original research presented by an organization or researcher; 2) eyewitness accounts of events, personal experience, or work experience; 3) first-person editorials offering pundits' opinions; 4) government officials presenting political plans and/or policies; 5) representatives of organizations presenting testimony or policy.

❝Tumors have the potential to arise from any of the diverse cells and tissue types that normally occur within the brain or spinal cord; in some cases, tumors will develop from a combination of cell or tissue types.❞

—American Association for Cancer Research, "Brain and Spinal Cord Cancer," July 17, 2008. www.aacr.org.

The American Association for Cancer Research is an organization that seeks to prevent and cure cancer through research, education, communication, and collaboration.

❝Tumors can be classified as benign or malignant. Benign tumors are usually those that remain well encapsulated without the ability to spread either locally or to distant sites.❞

—Children's Hospital Boston, "Brain Tumors," January 25, 2010. www.childrenshospital.org.

Children's Hospital Boston is one of the largest pediatric medical centers in the United States.

❝Symptoms are often vague in children, especially in very young children who are not able to fully describe their symptoms. Some of these symptoms can occur with a variety of more common childhood illnesses.❞

—National Brain Tumor Society, "Brain Tumor FAQ," 2010. www.braintumor.org.

The National Brain Tumor Society exists to find a cure and improve the quality of life for those who are affected by brain tumors.

❝Because the brain and spinal cord are enclosed in rigid containers (skull and spine), abnormal growths may be noticed simply because there is not enough room for them.❞

—Children's Brain Tumor Foundation, "What Is a Tumor, and What Makes Brain Tumors Different from Other Tumors?" November 10, 2009. www.cbtf.org.

The Children's Brain Tumor Foundation supports children with brain and spinal cord tumors and their families.

❝It is not very common for cancers to spread to the brain, but it can happen.❞

—Cancer Research UK, "Where a Cancer Spreads," March 26, 2010. www.cancerhelp.org.uk.

Cancer Research UK is a research organization based in London that is dedicated to preventing, diagnosing, and treating cancer.

❝Brain tumors do not discriminate. Primary brain tumors—those that begin in the brain and tend to stay in the brain—occur in people of all ages, but they are statistically more frequent in children and older adults.❞

—American Brain Tumor Association, "Facts & Statistics," 2010. www.abta.org.

The American Brain Tumor Association provides research funding for brain tumor diagnosis, treatment, and care, with the ultimate goal of finding a cure.

What Are Brain Tumors?

- According to the Brain Science Foundation, more than **612,000** people are living with primary brain tumors in the United States.

- Krebsliga Schweiz (the Swiss Cancer League) states that an average of **1 in 10,000** adults and **1 in 50,000** children worldwide suffer from a brain tumor.

- The National Institute of Neurological Disorders and Stroke states that more than **195,000** Americans are diagnosed with a brain tumor each year.

- According to University Hospital in Newark, New Jersey, malignant brain tumors make up only about **1.3 percent** of all cancers in the United States.

- The U.S. Central Brain Tumor Registry states that **62,930** new cases of primary nonmalignant and malignant brain and spinal cord tumors were expected to be diagnosed in the United States in 2010.

- The Memorial Sloan-Kettering Cancer Center states that about **100,000** people in the United States are diagnosed with brain metastases (cancers that have spread from other parts of the body) each year.

- The National Brain Tumor Society states that gliomas (tumors arising from the brain's supportive tissue) represent **32 percent** of all brain tumors and **80 percent** of those that are malignant.

Most Common Childhood Cancers

Malignant tumors of the central nervous system (including the brain) are the second most common form of cancer in children, surpassed only by leukemia. A study published in the June 2008 issue of *Pediatrics* examined all the various cancers that affect children and youth aged 19 and under, and some of the most common types are shown in this graph.

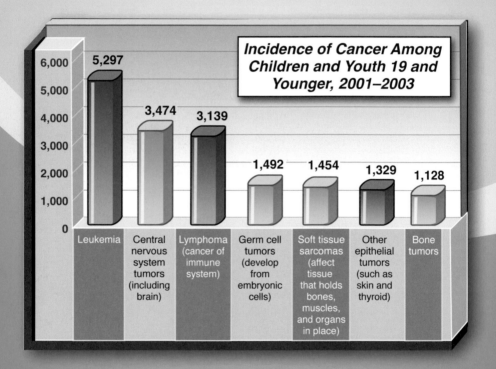

Incidence of Cancer Among Children and Youth 19 and Younger, 2001–2003

Source: Jun Li et al., "Cancer Incidence Among Children and Adolescents in the United States, 2001–2003," *Pediatrics*, June 2008. http://pediatrics.aapublications.org.

- According to Children's Hospital Boston, approximately **2,200** children and adolescents in the United States are diagnosed with a brain tumor each year.

The Brain and Its Functions

Although the human brain weighs only about 3 pounds, it controls everything from breathing and moving to learning, thinking, and remembering. This illustration shows the functions of the different areas of a healthy human brain. How severely one or more of these functions are impaired by a brain tumor depends on its size, type, and location.

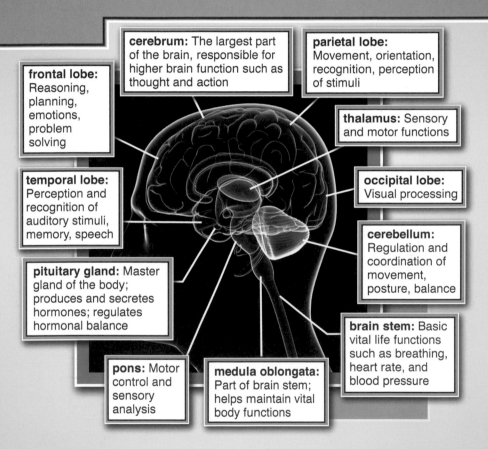

cerebrum: The largest part of the brain, responsible for higher brain function such as thought and action

parietal lobe: Movement, orientation, recognition, perception of stimuli

frontal lobe: Reasoning, planning, emotions, problem solving

thalamus: Sensory and motor functions

temporal lobe: Perception and recognition of auditory stimuli, memory, speech

occipital lobe: Visual processing

cerebellum: Regulation and coordination of movement, posture, balance

pituitary gland: Master gland of the body; produces and secretes hormones; regulates hormonal balance

brain stem: Basic vital life functions such as breathing, heart rate, and blood pressure

pons: Motor control and sensory analysis

medula oblongata: Part of brain stem; helps maintain vital body functions

Source: Serendip (Bryn Mawr College), "Brain Structures and Their Functions," June 3, 2005. http://serendip.brynmawr.edu.

- According to the Memorial Sloan-Kettering Cancer Center, metastatic brain cancer (cancer that spreads from another part of the body) is about **10 times** more common than cancer that starts in the brain.

Brain Tumor Warning Signs

The symptoms of brain tumors vary based on the type, size, and location. This list shows some of the most common symptoms for someone with a secondary (metastatic) brain tumor, or one that has spread to the brain from cancer elsewhere in the body. According to the National Institutes of Health, metastatic brain tumors are much more common than primary brain tumors, which originate in the brain.

Symptoms of Metastatic Brain Tumors

- Decreased coordination, clumsiness, falls
- Rapid emotional changes, strange behaviors
- Fever (occasional)
- Lethargy, general ill feelings
- Headache—recent or a new onset of more severe headaches than usual
- Memory loss, poor judgement, difficulty solving problems
- Numbness, tingling, pain, and other changes in sensation
- Personality changes
- Seizures—new for the person
- Speech difficulties
- Vision changes, such as double vision or decreased vision
- Vomiting, with or without nausea
- Weakness of a body area

Source: National Institutes of Health, "Metastatic Brain Tumor," MedLine Plus, March 2, 2010. www.nlm.nih.gov.

- According to the Memorial Sloan-Kettering Cancer Center, malignant melanoma (a malignancy of pigment-producing cells located primarily in the skin) is responsible for nearly **50 percent** of brain cancer cases.

What Causes Brain Tumors?

66Little is known about the causes of primary brain tumours.99

—Krebsliga Schweiz (Swiss Cancer League), which supports cancer research and seeks to increase public awareness of cancer prevention measures.

66Although we do not know why one person gets brain cancer while another does not, we know it is not caused by drinking alcohol during pregnancy, watching television, drinking diet sodas or not eating enough vegetables.99

—Children's Hospital Boston, which is one of the largest pediatric medical centers in the United States.

One of the most difficult tasks for doctors is having to tell a patient that he or she has a brain tumor. The announcement is typically met with a reaction of shock, followed by the inevitable questions: "How did this happen? What caused it?" Unfortunately, even the most renowned brain experts cannot provide the answers that patients seek because no one knows, with any certainty, what causes brain tumors. As New York neurosurgeon John R. Mangiardi writes:

> Scientists, physicians and researchers ponder the limitless questions concerning brain tumors: What does a brain tumor eat for breakfast? How does it really function? Why can't we get rid of this thing now? Why did person A get a brain tumor and not B? What causes brain

tumors? These are just a few of the hundreds of questions plaguing scientists, researchers, as well as patients, their families and their physicians.[28]

The Genetics Connection

Many diseases and disorders are known to be hereditary. This is true of congenital heart disease, some types of cancer, schizophrenia, and cystic fibrosis, among others. But heredity is not usually a factor in the development of brain tumors, as the National Cancer Institute explains: "It is rare for brain tumors to run in a family. Only a very small number of families have several members with brain tumors."[29] There are, however, certain genetic disorders that increase the risk for someone to develop a brain tumor. One such condition is neurofibromatosis, which is characterized by the growth of benign tumors known as neurofibromas. The tumors can grow in any area of the body where there are nerve cells, including the spinal cord and brain.

> **According to the National Institute on Deafness and Other Communication Disorders, patients with neurofibromatosis type 2 often develop multiple tumors of the brain and spinal cord, and these tumors can become life threatening as they grow.**

A rare form of this disorder, neurofibromatosis type 2 (NF2), is associated with tumors known as bilateral vestibular schwannomas, which develop from an overproduction of Schwann cells in the brain. According to the National Institute on Deafness and Other Communication Disorders, patients with neurofibromatosis type 2 often develop multiple tumors of the brain and spinal cord, and these tumors can become life threatening as they grow. Tumors can also develop on nerves that are essential for swallowing, speech, eye and facial movement, and facial sensation.

Another tumor-producing genetic disorder is tuberous sclerosis, which has also been linked to brain tumors. The National Institute of Neurological Disorders and Stroke says that tuberous sclerosis commonly affects the central nervous system and can result in tumors of the brain, as well as other vital organs such as the kidneys, heart, and lungs. Three types of brain tumors have been associated with tuberous sclerosis. One, known as a cortical tuber, usually forms on the brain's surface but may also appear in deeper areas of the brain. Tumors known as subependymal nodules form on the walls of the brain's ventricles, while astrocytomas can form in various parts of the central nervous system.

Radiation Exposure

Studies have shown that people who have been exposed to radiation have a higher risk of developing primary brain tumors than the general population. This is especially true if the radiation exposure occurred at a young age, such as someone who was treated with high-dose radiation therapy as a child and develops a malignant brain tumor as an adult. Christopher Dolinsky writes: "Higher radiation doses are generally felt to increase the risk of eventually developing a brain tumor, and radiation-induced brain tumors can take anywhere from 10–30 years to form."[30]

The reason radiation therapy is a risk factor for brain tumors is that radiation kills not only cancerous cells, but also healthy brain cells. The American Cancer Society explains: "In a child, healthy cells in the bone, brain, and other organs, are growing fast. . . . Treatment can damage these cells and keep them from growing and developing the way they should."[31] Radiation treatment involves the use of high-energy rays to kill cancer cells and shrink tumors. The radiation doses are directly correlated with a patient's risk for brain tumors later in life, meaning that the higher the dose, the greater the risk that a primary brain tumor will develop.

This was a concern expressed by a man named Dave Embrey, who posted on an online cancer forum. In March 2010 his mother was diagnosed with an astrocytoma inside her brain stem. Embrey noted that when she was a child, she underwent radiation therapy for a cancerous brain tumor, and it went away. The woman's new tumor is very close to the location of the old one, and her symptoms are similar to those she suffered as a child: daily headaches, double vision, only partial movement in one eye, and balance problems. Embrey asks: "Is it possible that this tumor is caused by radiation from 53 years ago?"[32] Many brain cancer specialists say that this sort of recurrence is indeed possible.

Toxic Substances and Brain Tumors

Whether exposure to chemicals raises the risk of developing a brain tumor is of interest to scientists. Laboratory experiments have shown that certain industrial chemicals cause brain tumors in mice. Some chemicals that have been tested include organic solvents; vinyl chloride, which is used to make plastics; and N-nitroso compounds, which are used by tanneries, pesticide manufacturers, dye-making plants, foundries, and rubber manufacturers. But, as Dolinsky writes, "when examining populations exposed to these various chemicals (like pesticide workers or workers in the petrochemical industry), there has never been any conclusive evidence to suggest that they get brain tumors at a higher rate than people without the chemical exposures."[33]

Although a link between chemical exposure and human brain tumors has not been proved, some people are convinced that there *is* a connection—especially those who say they have personally been affected by it. This has been a source of heated controversy among residents of a sprawling residential development in southern Florida known as The Acreage. Between 1994 and 2008, children and/or teenagers from 13 families living in the area were diagnosed with brain tumors or cancer of the central nervous system. Because of the unusually high number of illnesses, Florida health officials designated The Acreage as a cancer cluster, which is defined by the National Cancer Institute as the occurrence of a larger-than-expected number of cases of cancer within a group of people in a geographic area over a period of time.

> **The reason radiation therapy is a risk factor for brain tumors is that radiation kills not only cancerous cells, but also healthy brain cells.**

Some of the families whose children developed brain tumors are convinced that a nearby defense contractor, Pratt and Whitney, is responsible for the cancer cluster. Over the years, the company has had a number of toxic waste spills at its site. In spite of these spills, Pratt and Whitney officials insist that there has been little or no leakage into groundwater. But tests have shown that the area's groundwater contains toxic substances such as petroleum, various heavy metals, and dioxane, a chemical that is used as a solvent.

Although no definitive link has been found between the elevated cases of brain tumors and polluted groundwater, scientists agree that more testing needs to be done. But since the possibility exists, and such an unusually high number of young people have become ill, many residents are fearful and are considering moving away from the area. Tracy Newfield, whose teenage daughter Jessica developed a malignant brain tumor five years ago, is one of them. She shares her thoughts: "I have to . . . make sure I can look at my daughter and say, 'I don't think it's an environmental cause.' I don't feel that right now."[34]

> " Although a link between chemical exposure and human brain tumors has not been proved, some people are convinced that there *is* a connection—especially those who say they have personally been affected by it. "

Clues About Brain Metastases

Scientists have long known that metastatic tumors are caused by cancer that spreads to the brain from other parts of the body, but the process by which this occurs is not well understood. In an effort to learn more about how metastases work, a team of researchers from Oxford University in England performed a study that focused on how tumors grow in the brain—and what they discovered may someday improve survival rates for people with brain cancer.

The team analyzed a wide range of malignant cell types, including cells from melanoma, breast cancer, and lymphoma, a cancer that affects the immune system. They injected cancerous cells into the bloodstream of mice, and several days later they examined the creatures' brains. The researchers found that in 95 percent of cases, the cells had attached themselves to the walls of blood vessels in the brain, rather than to brain cells. This was an indication that cancer cells latch onto the brain's blood vessels and are able to get all the nutrients and oxygen they need to grow.

Another finding was that a type of protein called integrin plays an essential role in the ability of cancerous cells to adhere to blood vessels. Integrin exists on the outside surface of cancer cells. When the researchers removed the protein, the cells were no longer able to stick to blood vessels, and their growth stopped. Ruth Muschel, who led the research team, explains the significance of this discovery: "Our research describes a novel mechanism which explains how tumour cells metastasize to the brain. The dependency of early brain metastases on the host blood vessels might provide a target for new drug therapies."[35]

The Cell Phone Controversy

One of the most hotly debated topics about primary brain tumors is whether they can be caused by heavy cell phone use. Cell phones emit a form of electromagnetic radiation known as radio-frequency energy. When the phones are held up to the ear, the radiation is emitted close to the brain. The potential danger of this was the subject of an analysis performed by Vini Khurana, a neurosurgeon from Australia. Khurana spent 15 months reviewing more than 100 studies on the effects of cell phones and determined that people who use them for 10 years or more can double their risk of developing brain cancer. At the conclusion of the study, Khurana stated that "this danger has far broader public health ramifications than asbestos and smoking, and directly concerns all of us, particularly the younger generation, including very young children."[36]

> " One of the most hotly debated topics about primary brain tumors is whether they can be caused by heavy cell phone use. "

To perform an in-depth examination of the possible link between cell phone use and brain tumors, the International Agency for Research on Cancer commissioned a long-term study that was released in May 2010. Known as Interphone, the study group was composed of 21 international scientists. It involved nearly 13,000 participants from 13 countries, including 2,708 who suffered from glioma, 2,409 with meningioma, and 1,200 with other types of tumors. The remaining participants, who were matched to the others by age, sex, and region, made up the control group. After the study was concluded, the agency's director, Christopher Wild, stated: "An increased risk of brain cancer is not established from the data from Interphone."[37]

There were, however, some findings that many insist must not be overlooked. For instance, the investigators found that 10 percent of people who used their cell phones often and for the longest period of time (30 minutes or more of calls per day) had a significantly higher risk of developing some form of brain cancer than those in the control group. Another discovery was a higher-than-normal incidence of gliomas among heavy cell phone users.

Siegal Sadetzki, a physician from Israel, was part of the Interphone study group. She acknowledges that the study did not definitively confirm an association between cell phones and brain tumors—but neither did it dismiss a possible link. She explains:

> We do see a few indications of risk. And these indications appear among people who were exposed for the longest duration. We do see an association with ipsilateral use [tumors on the same side of the head that a user holds a cell phone to the ear]. We also see an association with temporal lobe [brain] exposure. So there are some indications of a positive association in these subgroups. . . . We do have some suspicions.[38]

Because the Interphone study leaves many unanswered questions, Sadetzki and other like-minded scientists agree that further research is necessary.

Questions Linger

Brain tumors are mysterious for many reasons, and much about their cause remains unknown. Many theories exist, from high-dose radiation and toxic chemical exposure to radio-frequency energy emitted by cell phones. As scientists continue to study brain tumors, they will make additional discoveries and undoubtedly learn more about potential causes. Perhaps this will lead to a time in the future when patients diagnosed with brain tumors no longer have to hear that the cause is unknown.

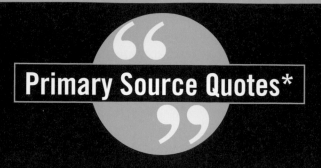

Primary Source Quotes*

What Causes Brain Tumors?

66 Studies have shown a correlation between the side that a patient uses their cell phone and the side of the brain where their glioblastoma occurs, a correlation I've noticed in a great many of my patients. 99

—Keith Black, *Brain Surgeon*. New York: Wellness Central-Hatchett Book Group, 2009.

Black is a neurosurgeon who is director of the Maxine Dunitz Neurosurgical Institute at Cedars-Sinai Medical Center in Los Angeles.

66 The use of cell phones has NOT been linked to an increased incidence of brain cancers. 99

—National Institutes of Health, "X-Plain Brain Tumors: Reference Summary," National Library of Medicine, Medline Plus, April 30, 2008. www.nlm.nih.gov.

The National Institutes of Health is the leading medical research agency in the United States.

Bracketed quotes indicate conflicting positions.

* Editor's Note: While the definition of a primary source can be narrowly or broadly defined, for the purposes of Compact Research, a primary source consists of: 1) results of original research presented by an organization or researcher; 2) eyewitness accounts of events, personal experience, or work experience; 3) first-person editorials offering pundits' opinions; 4) government officials presenting political plans and/or policies; 5) representatives of organizations presenting testimony or policy.

❝Primary brain tumors begin when normal cells acquire errors (mutations) in their DNA. These mutations allow cells to grow and divide at increased rates and to continue living when healthy cells would die.❞

—Mayo Clinic, "Brain Tumor," May 15, 2010. www.mayoclinic.com.

The Mayo Clinic is a world-renowned medical facility headquartered in Rochester, Minnesota.

....

❝There is no known behavioral or environmental factor that leads to brain tumors. Fears about cellular phones, microwave ovens, foods or food additives, and other rumored brain carcinogens have no scientific basis.❞

—Lisa M. DeAngelis, "Brain Tumors—The Dana Guide," Dana Foundation, *The Dana Guide to Brain Health*, June 2009. www.dana.org.

DeAngelis is chair of the Department of Neurology at the Memorial Sloan-Kettering Cancer Center.

....

❝No one knows the exact cause of brain tumors, yet they are the leading cause of solid-tumor death in children . . . and now the second-fastest growing reason for cancer death among those over age 65.❞

—American Brain Tumor Association, "About Brain Tumors," 2010. www.abta.org.

The American Brain Tumor Association provides research funding for brain tumor diagnosis, treatment, and care, with the ultimate goal of finding a cure.

....

❝For primary brain tumors, two environmental risk factors are exposure of the head to Xrays and a history of disorders of the immune system. Certain genetic disorders present risk factors for specific types of brain tumors, both cancerous and noncancerous.❞

—Brain Science Foundation, "Frequently Asked Questions," 2010. www.brainsciencefoundation.org.

The Brain Science Foundation seeks to increase awareness of primary brain tumors and to make brain tumor research a priority.

....

❝Today we know much more than we did even 5 years ago about genetic and cellular alterations that may cause brain tumors.❞

—Elizabeth M. Wilson, preface to *100 Questions & Answers About Brain Tumors*, by Virginia Stark-Vance and M.L. Dubay. Sudbury, MA: Jones and Bartlett, 2011.

Wilson is executive director of the American Brain Tumor Association.

❝Taking the still relatively short time for use of wireless phones on a broad scale . . . the results showing increasing brain tumour incidence may be early warning of future public health problems.❞

—Lennart Hardell and Michael Carlberg, "Mobile Phones, Cordless Phones and the Risk for Brain Tumours," *International Journal of Oncology*, July 2009.

Hardell and Carlberg are with the department of oncology at Örebro University Hospital in Örebro, Sweden.

❝Cancer cells can break away from the primary tumor site and travel through blood and lymphatic vessels. This is how cancer cells spread, or metastasize, to another part of the body, such as the brain.❞

—Memorial Sloan-Kettering Cancer Center, "Brain Tumors, Metastatic: Overview," April 28, 2009. www.mskcc.org.

The Memorial Sloan-Kettering Cancer Center is a world-renowned cancer facility that is headquartered in New York City.

What Causes Brain Tumors?

- **Age** is a factor in the development of brain tumors; according to the American Brain Tumor Association, the lowest incidence is among young people aged 20 and younger, with the risk steadily increasing each year.

- The National Cancer Institute states that brain tumors are **rarely hereditary**, with only a small number of families having several members with brain tumors.

- According to Children's Hospital Boston, most pediatric brain tumors are caused by **mutations** in several genes.

- The American Cancer Society states that radiation from **high-dose X-rays** can cause cell damage that leads to a brain tumor.

- According to a study published in 2009 by Swedish researchers, after one or more years of cell phone use, the risk of brain cancer in people who begin using cell phones before they turn 20 is **5.2 times greater** than for the general population.

- The wireless telephone trade organization CTIA states that as of December 2009 there were **285 million** cell phones in use in the United States, covering **91 percent** of the population.

Risk Factors for Brain Tumors

Scientists do not know what causes primary brain tumors, which are those that originate in the brain. Potential risk factors include genetics, exposure to chemicals or radiation, and age.

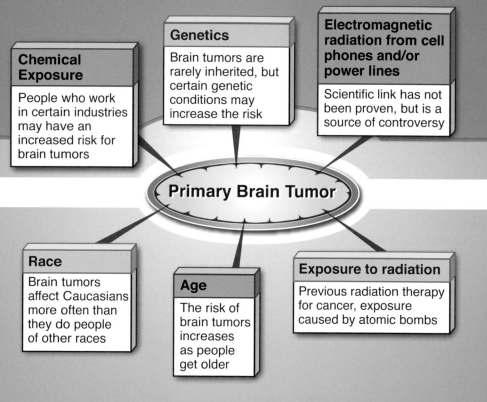

Chemical Exposure

People who work in certain industries may have an increased risk for brain tumors

Genetics

Brain tumors are rarely inherited, but certain genetic conditions may increase the risk

Electromagnetic radiation from cell phones and/or power lines

Scientific link has not been proven, but is a source of controversy

Primary Brain Tumor

Race

Brain tumors affect Caucasians more often than they do people of other races

Age

The risk of brain tumors increases as people get older

Exposure to radiation

Previous radiation therapy for cancer, exposure caused by atomic bombs

Source: Mayo Clinic, "Brain Tumor," May 15, 2010. www.mayoclinic.com.

- According to the American Brain Tumor Association, **ethnicity** is a factor in the development of brain tumors; the overall incidence rate for primary brain tumors is 17.73 per 100,000 for Hispanics, compared to 19.13 per 100,000 for non-Hispanic whites.

- The Mayo Clinic states that people working in **chemical industries** have an increased risk of developing brain tumors.

Cell Phones and Brain Tumors

Whether heavy use of cell phones contributes to the development of brain tumors has been the subject of numerous studies, and is a highly controversial issue. In 2010 a Kansas newspaper conducted a poll asking readers if they believed there was a connection between brain cancer and cell phones and 46 percent of them said no.

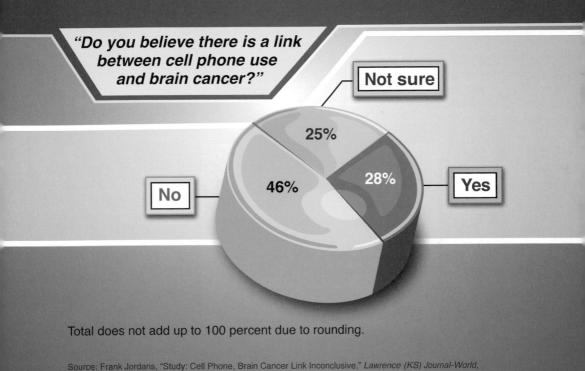

"Do you believe there is a link between cell phone use and brain cancer?"

Not sure 25%

No 46%

Yes 28%

Total does not add up to 100 percent due to rounding.

Source: Frank Jordans, "Study: Cell Phone, Brain Cancer Link Inconclusive," *Lawrence (KS) Journal-World*, May 17, 2010. www2.ljworld.com.

- According to New York neurosurgeon John R. Mangiardi, brain tumors in children most often result from **immature or primitive cells** that are still developing and have not reached full maturity.

- Children's Hospital Boston states that children who have received **radiation to the head** as part of prior treatment for other cancers are at risk for new brain tumors later in life.

Cancer That Spreads to the Brain

Although scientists do not know what causes primary brain tumors (which originate in the brain), the cause of metastatic brain tumors is better understood. These tumors develop when malignant cells from cancer elsewhere in the body break off from the main cancer site, travel through the bloodstream, and lodge in the brain. Many types of cancer can spread, but according to the National Institutes of Health, some of the most common are cancer of the lung, breast, kidney, and testis, as well as melanoma.

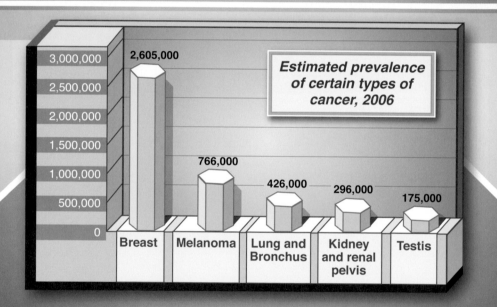

Estimated prevalence of certain types of cancer, 2006

	Breast	Melanoma	Lung and Bronchus	Kidney and renal pelvis	Testis
	2,605,000	766,000	426,000	296,000	175,000

Source: American Cancer Society, "Cancer Prevalence: How Many People Have Cancer?" 2009. www.cancer.org.

- According to the Mayo Clinic, secondary brain tumors most often occur in people who have a **history of cancer**.

- The American Cancer Society states that certain genetic conditions such as **neurofibromatosis** and **tuberous sclerosis** (both of which involve the growth of tumors in the body) have been linked with the development of brain tumors.

What Are the Risks of Brain Tumors?

> **Perhaps no other cancer is as feared as brain tumor since severe disability, including paralysis, seizures, gait disturbances, and impairment of intellectual capacity may occur.**
>
> —J. Stephen Huff, an emergency medicine and neurology professor at the University of Virginia's Department of Emergency Medicine.

> **Depending on the type, a growing tumor can kill healthy cells or disrupt their function. It can move or press on sensitive tissue and block the flow of blood and other fluid, causing pain and inflammation.**
>
> —National Institute for Neurological Disorders and Stroke, which seeks to reduce the burden of neurological disease throughout the world with research and education.

The clival chordoma is among the deadliest of all brain tumors. It develops in the clivus, a bone in the base of the skull that is close to the brain stem and carotid arteries, two large blood vessels that supply blood to the brain. Although clival chordomas are often benign, they are aggressive tumors that push their way into adjacent tissues and disrupt vital function of the brain stem. Neurologist Martin L. Lazar writes: "In spite of modern treatment, local recurrence of this tumor results in local destruction of vital neural structures which eventually is the cause of death."[39]

Gerard Kelly, a man from a small town near Dublin, Ireland, was diagnosed with a clival chordoma when he was 25 years old. Neurosurgeons had removed it during one operation, but as these tumors often do, it grew back. The surgeons tried a second time but were able to get only a small portion of the newly grown tumor out. They told Kelly there was nothing more that could be done, and he only had a few more months to live. Frightened but not willing to give up, Kelly and his brother made the long trip to Los Angeles, California, to visit Dr. Keith Black at Cedars-Sinai Medical Center. Black writes: "He looked at me as if I was his last hope."[40]

Enemy of the Brain

Black was stunned when he reviewed Kelly's MRI scans, declaring the tumor to be the largest clival chordoma that he had ever seen. He called it "a vast, hydra-headed monster,"[41] referring to Hydra, a ferocious, many-headed beast of Greek mythology that grew two new heads whenever one was chopped off. And even though the tumor was benign, it was indeed a formidable beast. Much of its ability to spread was due to a previous surgery, during which the doctor had cut through Kelly's dura mater, the protective covering of the brain beneath the skull. In doing that, Black writes, "he had set the ogre loose. No longer sandwiched between the dura and the skull, the unfettered clival chordoma had mushroomed as it grew into the breach."[42]

> " Although clival chordomas are often benign, they are aggressive tumors that push their way into adjacent tissues and disrupt vital function of the brain stem. "

Once Kelly's tumor had pushed through the dura mater, it moved into his brain, coiled itself around the brain stem, and squeezed major arteries and surrounding blood vessels by encircling them. From there the tumor kept spreading, embedding itself in the spine and creeping down to the third cervical vertebra, one of the bones in the upper part of the neck.

By the time Kelly sought help from Black, the tumor had taken over his brain to the extent that he was nearly incapacitated. He was extremely weak, and due to compression on his brain stem and nerves, he was having vision problems and difficulty maintaining his balance. His hearing had deteriorated, and with the tumor pressing on his vocal cords, it was extremely hard for him to speak. Because he was no longer able to swallow, a feeding tube had been implanted in his stomach.

During two separate operations, Black was able to remove 95 percent of the tumor, leaving a piece about the size of half a pencil eraser. The tiny remnant was trapped by scar tissue in the lower part of the brain stem, and Black could not remove it without causing severe neurological damage. With the fragment still embedded in Kelly's brain, Black knew that it was only a matter of time before the tumor grew back. His hope was that it would grow away from the brain stem rather than toward it, and if so, Kelly would likely live for several more years. Unfortunately, though, that was not what happened.

> " According to the American Brain Tumor Association, mass effect can damage the brain by compressing and displacing delicate brain tissue. "

As Black had feared it might, the tumor grew into Kelly's brain stem, where it compressed the delicate nerve pathways that directed all of his body's functions. A little more than six months after he and his brother returned to Ireland, Kelly became ill with pneumonia, lost most of the feeling in his body, and died shortly afterward. Upon hearing the news, Black was devastated, but he knew he had done everything possible to save his patient. He writes: "Was Gerard Kelly's surgery worth it? Absolutely. . . . It was very clear that this young man and his family, even if the chances were very small, wanted at least the opportunity to survive."[43]

Risks for Children

Just as tumors (both benign and malignant) can severely damage the brains of adults, the same is true in children. In fact, because their young brains have not fully developed, tumors can be even more damaging to children, sometimes causing life-threatening problems. One of the most common risks is the buildup of cerebrospinal fluid in the brain, which is a condition known as hydrocephalus. John R. Mangiardi writes: "The entire brain floats in a self contained sort of womb, and like a fetus, is surrounded by and filled with a watery fluid known as cerebrospinal fluid (CSF). These fluid spaces, when obstructed by a tumor, may enlarge and cause pressure within the closed box of the hard skull to increase dangerously. This is referred to as hydrocephalus or water-on-the-brain."[44] According to University of Virginia physician J. Stephen Huff, if a ventricle that usually drains cerebrospinal fluid remains obstructed, the child is at risk of immediate death.

> "When people have seizures of any type, they may lose control of their actions and become injured by falling or hitting things around them."

The intense pressure that is caused by hydrocephalus, as well as a tumor growing within the tight confines of the skull, can lead to what is known as mass effect. According to the American Brain Tumor Association, mass effect can damage the brain by compressing and displacing delicate brain tissue. Children who sustain this sort of brain damage are at risk for developing neurological problems such as learning disabilities. The Children's Brain Tumor Foundation explains: "Unfortunately, survivors of childhood brain tumors frequently develop problems in the areas of intellectual ability, academic achievement, memory, and attention. . . . Learning disabilities are particularly common among brain tumor survivors, and many children with learning disabilities require special education services at school."[45] The group adds that children may also develop impaired vision as a result of a brain tumor, as well as hearing deficiencies.

The Danger of Seizures

Of all the symptoms exhibited by people with brain tumors, seizures are among the most common. In fact, they may be one of the first symptoms to appear. Seizures are an indication of abnormal electrical activity in the brain, as the American Brain Tumor Association explains: "It is similar to seeing a circuit breaker trip during an electrical power storm. Normally, your body's nerve cells communicate with each other via carefully controlled 'electric' signals. Those nerve cells send thousands of signals back and forth, giving instructions to all parts of the body. If something interferes with those signals and they become more intense, a seizure results."[46]

Depending on the tumor's rate of growth, seizures may be present for a long period of time before a brain tumor is diagnosed. They may also continue for months or even years after treatment has been complete. In some cases seizures can cause brain damage, as Duke University neurologist Mohamad Mikati explains: "If seizures are not controlled, especially if they are frequent and violent, they can injure the brain."[47]

> " Sometimes the psychological pain is as difficult for brain tumor patients as their physical suffering. "

Seizures can create risky situations for those who suffer from them. This is true not only of the most severe tonic clonic seizures, but also what are known as absence seizures. Those who experience absence seizures may seem to have zoned out momentarily, staring off into space with a blank look on their faces. These seizures appear to be mild, but, as the Mayo Clinic states, "that doesn't mean they can't be dangerous."[48]

When people have seizures of any type, they may lose control of their actions and become injured by falling or hitting things around them. If a seizure happens while someone is swimming, he or she is in danger of drowning. Studies have shown that people who suffer from recurrent seizures have a much higher risk of drowning than the general population. Other potential threats include vehicle accidents if people have seizures while driving, choking if a seizure occurs while eating, or severe burns if someone has a seizure while standing near a stove or campfire.

A Teen's Painful Struggle

Many problems that are associated with brain tumors can be serious, and often life threatening. But sometimes the psychological pain is as difficult for brain tumor patients as their physical suffering. For Katie Rozenas, a teenager from Massachusetts, the emotional pain was more traumatic than the physical effects of her illness. She shares how she felt when doctors gave her the diagnosis: "'You have a brain tumor and the only solution is brain surgery to remove it.' Imagine hearing that when you're 16 years old and have never broken anything and have only gone to the hospital two or three times in your life. That was my reality in March of 2008."[49]

In some ways the months before the diagnosis were even more difficult. Rozenas experienced an unexplainable weight gain during her junior year of high school. She joined a weight loss program and spent an hour or two each day running on a treadmill, but the pounds continued to pile on. It was hard enough for her to look in the mirror and see a body that she no longer recognized—but when she became the object of ridicule at school, she was crushed. She writes:

> The most painful thing was what my weight gain caused people in and out of school to say about me. . . . My classmates said things like, 'I don't blame her for not wanting to go swimming. If I was like her, I wouldn't either' and 'What, does she have diabetes?' and 'Look at that girl, she's such a chunky monkey.' It got to the point where I didn't eat or jump or run in front of people. I knew people were talking about me behind my back. . . . I tried to keep my head up, but it was hard when I felt like the world was against me and time was passing me by.[50]

Finally after a series of tests, a specialist at Children's Hospital Boston discovered the problem. Rozenas suffered from Cushing's disease, an illness that is so rare it only strikes about 1 in 10 million young people. Cushing's, which is characterized by obesity and an inability to lose weight, is caused by a benign tumor on the pituitary gland. The master gland of the body, the pea-sized pituitary gland is located at the base of the brain behind the eyes. It produces and secretes many types of hormones, as well as regulates the body's hormonal balance. Because of the tumor—which was no larger than a grain of rice—Rozenas's hormones were thrown out of balance, and that is what caused her extreme weight gain.

She underwent surgery in May 2008 to have the tumor removed. Almost immediately after surgery, her hormones began to level out, and she started to lose the weight she had gained. Today she is back to her normal size and feels like she has her life back. But the ordeal gave her some insight that she did not have before, as she explains: "I don't want people to feel sorry for me. I just want them to take from my story this moral and treat other people better. I have eyes that are less judgmental and a mind that is more open. When someone [who is overweight] walks by me I think maybe it's not their fault. And that is one thing many people, not only 16 year olds, don't think about as they go through life."[51]

"Life Can Change You"

Numerous risks are associated with brain tumors, whether they are benign or malignant. Some, like clival chordomas, can weave their way through a person's brain and squeeze the life out of the brain stem and critical arteries. Tumors can cause a dangerous buildup of cerebrospinal fluid in the brain, lead to seizures, or throw a person's whole system out of balance. As for how difficult living with a brain tumor can be, no one knows better than someone who has personally gone through it and survived the experience. Rozenas writes: "I've seen how quickly life can change. And how quickly life can change you."[52]

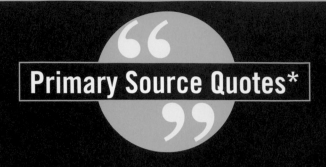

Primary Source Quotes*

What Are the Risks of Brain Tumors?

❝The brain is the one part of the body we cannot damage, cut out, or replace and still be ourselves.❞

—Keith Black, *Brain Surgeon*. New York: Wellness Central-Hatchett Book Group, 2009.

Black is a neurosurgeon who is director of the Maxine Dunitz Neurosurgical Institute at Cedars-Sinai Medical Center in Los Angeles.

❝The word 'benign' is misleading because it implies that the tumor presents no danger to the patient. In fact benign tumors of the central nervous system can cause very serious disability and even death.❞

—Brain Science Foundation, "Frequently Asked Questions," Primary Brain Tumors: An Information Clearinghouse, 2010. www.brainsciencefoundation.org.

The Brain Science Foundation seeks to increase awareness of primary brain tumors and to make brain tumor research a priority.

---

* Editor's Note: While the definition of a primary source can be narrowly or broadly defined, for the purposes of Compact Research, a primary source consists of: 1) results of original research presented by an organization or researcher; 2) eyewitness accounts of events, personal experience, or work experience; 3) first-person editorials offering pundits' opinions; 4) government officials presenting political plans and/or policies; 5) representatives of organizations presenting testimony or policy.

Primary Source Quotes

"Many children who are treated for brain tumors experience significant long-term problems, such as changes in intellectual and motor function."

—Children's Hospital Boston, "Brain Tumors," January 25, 2010. www.childrenshospital.org.

Children's Hospital Boston is one of the largest pediatric medical centers in the United States.

....

"A malignant tumor, also called 'cancer,' is always a threat to life. Malignant tumors invade and destroy healthy tissue. They usually grow rapidly, and can send 'roots' into normal tissue."

—Pediatric Brain Tumor Foundation, "How Pediatric Brain and Spinal Cord Tumors Are Diagnosed," 2010. www.pbtfus.org.

The Pediatric Brain Tumor Foundation advocates on behalf of children with brain tumors and their families by increasing public awareness and supporting medical research.

....

"Malignant gliomas still are dangerous and most patients will not survive them beyond a few years. Benign gliomas slowly grow, producing disabilities, and eventually are also fatal."

—Don M. Long, "Gliomas: The Latest Research," Dana Foundation, May 29, 2008. www.dana.org.

Long is a distinguished service professor in the neurology department at Johns Hopkins Hospital.

....

"Benign tumors can be dangerous because of their size and location, even though they may grow very slowly, displacing normal structures of the brain."

—Virginia Stark-Vance and M.L. Dubay, *100 Questions & Answers About Brain Tumors*. Sudbury, MA: Jones and Bartlett, 2011.

Stark-Vance is a physician who specializes in malignancies of the brain and spinal cord, and Dubay is a brain cancer survivor.

....

❝A tumor can cause damage by increasing pressure in the brain, by shifting the brain or pushing against the skull, and by invading and damaging nerves and healthy brain tissue.❞

—National Brain Tumor Society, "Brain Tumor FAQ," 2010. www.braintumor.org.

The National Brain Tumor Society exists to find a cure and improve the quality of life for those who are affected by brain tumors.

❝Cancer that starts in the brain rarely, if ever, spreads outside the brain. It can, however, spread further in the brain and cause disability and death.❞

—National Institutes of Health, "X-Plain Brain Tumors: Reference Summary," National Library of Medicine, Medline Plus, April 30, 2008. www.nlm.nih.gov.

The National Institutes of Health is the leading medical research agency in the United States.

What Are the Risks of Brain Tumors?

- **Brain tumors** are the most common of the solid tumors in children and the leading cause of death from solid tumors.

- The American Brain Tumor Association states that brain tumors are the second leading cause of **cancer-related deaths in children** after leukemia (cancer of the blood or bone marrow).

- A 2010 report by the American Cancer Society estimated that **13,140** people would die of cancer of the brain or nervous system that year.

- According to a 2010 study funded by the National Cancer Institute, childhood cancer survivors are **four times** more likely to develop **post-traumatic stress disorder** than the general population.

- The American Brain Tumor Association states that about **one-third** of people diagnosed with a brain tumor are not aware they have a tumor until they have a seizure.

- According to neurosurgeon Keith Black, **70 percent** of low-grade noncancerous tumors will eventually morph into higher-grade, more aggressive tumors.

- The Mayo Clinic states that a brain tumor that damages the nerves connected to the eyes or visual cortex (the part of the brain that produces visual information) can result in **double vision** or a **reduced field of vision**.

The Deadliest Cancers

All malignant tumors can be deadly, including those of the brain. But several other types of cancer are much more prevalent than brain cancer, and have significantly higher deaths.

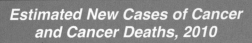

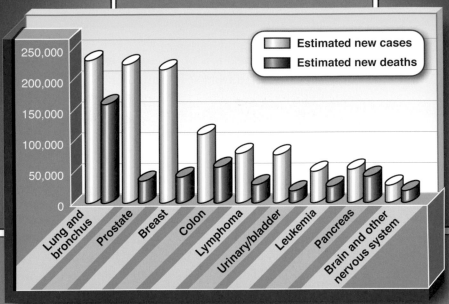

Estimated New Cases of Cancer and Cancer Deaths, 2010

Source: American Cancer Society, "Cancer Facts & Figures 2010," 2010. www.cancer.org.

- According to the American Brain Tumor Society, brain tumors are the **second** leading cause of cancer-related deaths in males up to age 39, and the **fifth** leading cause of cancer-related deaths in females aged 20 to 39.

- According to University of Virginia physician J. Stephen Huff, most patients with metastatic brain cancer die from the progression of their **primary cancer**, rather than from brain damage.

The Young Survive Longer

Brain cancer can be deadly for people of any age. But the five-year survival rate after someone is diagnosed with a malignant brain tumor decreases significantly with age.

Five-year survival rates after diagnosis of malignant tumor of the central nervous system (by age of diagnosis)

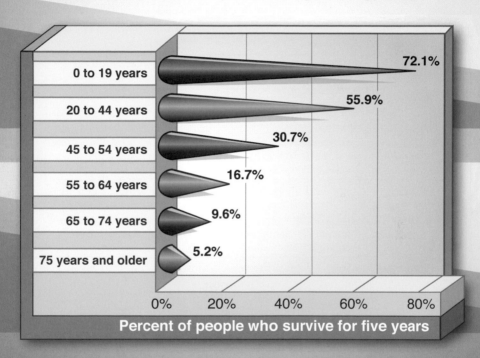

Source: Central Brain Tumor Registry of the United States, *CBTRUS Statistical Report: Primary Brain and Central Nervous System Tumors Diagnosed in the United States in 2004–2006*, February 2010. www.cbtrus.org.

- The Mayo Clinic states that the **weakness** caused by a brain tumor can be very similar to that caused by a stroke.

- According to New York neurosurgeon John R. Mangiardi, tumor cells always travel around the brain beyond the **tumor boundaries**, and can even be found on the opposite side of the brain.

Damage Caused by Brain Tumors

Tumors can harm the brain in a number of ways, depending on the type, location, and size. A tumor in the front of the parietal lobe, for example, may lead to numbness and impaired sensation, whereas a tumor on the left side of the temporal lobe may result in personality changes and impaired memory for words and language.

Frontal Lobe	
Back	Weakness and/or paralysis
Middle	Impaired ability to move the eyes and perform complex movements in the correct sequence
Front	Impaired concentration, reduced speech fluency, apathy; lack of inhibition can lead to socially inappropriate behavior
Parietal Lobe	
Back	Inability to distinguish right from left, problems with calculations and drawing
Front	Numbness, impaired sensation on opposite sides of body
Temporal Lobe	
Left side	Impaired memory for words and language, personality changes
Right side	Inability to do simple tasks, impaired memory for sounds and shapes
Occipital Lobe	
Front side	Difficulty recognizing familiar objects and faces and accurately interpreting what is seen
Both sides	People cannot see even though the eyes are functioning normally (known as cortical blindness)

Source: Merck, "Dysfunction by Location," *Merck Manual of Medical Information*, March 2008. www.merck.com.

- Brain tumors can cause women of childbearing age to stop having their **monthly periods** even though they are not pregnant.

How Successful Are Brain Tumor Treatments?

At his high school in Marietta, Georgia, Paul Amend was known as an outstanding student and a star athlete. Then at the beginning of his junior year, something strange began happening to him. He would be sitting at his desk in class, when suddenly it was like his brain switched off and the lights went out. After the moment passed, Amend felt confused, at first not realizing that he was in a classroom. His friend and football teammate Michael Abraham observed these episodes, as he explains: "Paul started zoning out every once in a while and it kind of got worse in time. He looked like he was in daze for about 20 seconds.

When he came to, he had lost track of time. He wasn't sure where he was or what was going on for a few seconds. It was scary."[53]

A Fighting Spirit

Amend remembered nothing of the blackouts except for what his teachers and classmates told him. He initially thought the episodes might be panic attacks, which he had experienced when he was in middle school, or perhaps the stress of academics combined with his heavy participation in three different sports. Finally, he acknowledged that something was wrong and told his parents. After several visits to doctors, Amend was diagnosed with a benign brain tumor known as an oligodendroglioma, which was about the size of a walnut. He learned that the blackouts had actually been absence seizures, a symptom of his tumor.

> " Although brain surgery has been performed for many years, technology now enables it to be more precise— and less risky— than ever before. "

In the fall of 2008, after football season had ended, Amend underwent surgery to have the tumor removed. Afterward he had what doctors call a remarkable recovery—by the following January he was again wrestling with his high school team, and he later also returned to playing lacrosse. He shares his thoughts about what he went through and his optimistic attitude about it: "I always looked at this as, This is another obstacle I have to deal with, this is the next part of my life. Everyone has a roadblock in their life; I just took mine as it came and embraced it."[54]

Surgical Removal

The type of treatment that is recommended for brain tumors varies depending on the size and type of the tumor, its rate of growth, and the general health of the patient. If it is determined that surgery would be safe, that is usually the first recommendation. Ideally, a surgeon will achieve what is known as a gross-total resection, meaning that the entire tumor has been removed. If that goal is accomplished, MRI scans taken after the operation should show no remaining signs of the tumor in the brain. This sort of surgery, whether a tumor is malignant or benign, is a delicate, specialized procedure that must be absolutely precise. Neurologist Don M. Long writes:

> Elsewhere in the body benign tumors can be cured by completely removing the tumor and, sometimes, a bit of the healthy tissue surrounding the tumor just to be sure. This does not often work for brain tumors for two reasons: In the brain, the location of the tumor often means even benign tumors cannot be removed without unacceptable damage to the patient. These tumors also infiltrate normal brain tissue; if all affected brain tissue were removed, the person would suffer severe neurological injury, making the cure as bad as the disease.[55]

The attempt to avoid severe neurological damage is why part of a tumor was left in 15-year-old Katie Proctor's brain. When she was a child, Katie underwent several operations for a brain stem glioma. Surgeons were able to remove 80 percent of the tumor, but a button-sized piece was embedded in her brain stem and could not be taken out—yet her brain was still irreparably damaged.

According to Katie's mother, Denni Proctor, the surgery left Katie deaf in her right ear and with limited vision in her right eye. One side of her face is paralyzed, which makes half of her mouth droop downward, and partial paralysis in her throat causes her to choke frequently when she is eating. She has periodic spells of vomiting that are sometimes so severe she needs to be hospitalized for dehydration. Proctor writes: "Her life will never be like a typical teenager's. Although she does a great job of making accommodations, Katie has issues every day of her life because of her brain tumor."[56]

Knives Without Blades

Although brain surgery has been performed for many years, technology now enables it to be more precise—and less risky—than ever before. One high-tech surgical tool is known as the Xknife, which kills tumor cells with X-ray beams. According to Keith Black, the instrument is similar to a large dental X-ray machine that rotates around the head and focuses X-ray beams at a particular point in the brain. The beams are precision-guided by an MRI scanner and a computer. Black writes: "Where the beams intersect, the dose of radiation is high enough to destroy all of the cancer, with minimal damage to surrounding healthy brain. The procedure is akin to burning a piece of paper with a magnifying glass, and has already shown great promise in dealing with metastatic tumors."[57]

Another high-tech surgical instrument is the gamma knife, which delivers more than 200 beams of radiation directly into a tumor with pinpoint accuracy. Because it can send the beams through a patient's intact skull, no surgical incisions are necessary. Gamma knife technology was first introduced in the 1980s but has been vastly improved over the years and is now highly sophisticated. According to the University of Maryland Medical Center, the procedure can stop tumors from growing in as much as 95 percent of all cases and also causes tumors to shrink in the majority of cases.

> **Because of the risks of radiation, some brain specialists are using a different type of treatment known as proton beam therapy.**

One of the patients for whom Black recommended the gamma knife procedure was Tionne Watkins. A well-known rhythm and blues/hip-hop star who goes by the name of T-Boz, Watkins had a brain tumor known as a vestibular schwannoma. It was growing on a nerve that is crucial for controlling hearing and balance and also affects the facial muscles. Watkins was terrified that her face would be paralyzed and that she would lose her hearing. Yet after gamma knife surgery, she experienced no problems. Black writes: "When Tionne woke up in Recovery, her facial muscles were working perfectly and she could hear. She had come through the surgery with no deficits. . . . The next day she was walking the halls."[58] Watkins fully recovered after the operation and returned to performing.

Minimally Invasive Surgery

Brain specialists have long known that brain operations in which the skull is cut open (known as craniotomies) carry serious potential risks for the patient. New York neurosurgeon Theodore H. Schwartz explains: "In traditional skull base surgery you have to open up the scalp and the head, move the brain aside, and manipulate the many nerves and arteries that are in the way to remove a tumor that sits at the very base of the skull—all of which can result in complications."[59] Avoiding potential brain damage is why many surgeons are turning to techniques that do not require making incisions in the scalp.

One such procedure, endoscopic brain surgery, involves reaching the tumor by going in through the nose or mouth. The technique was first described in the early twentieth century by an ear, nose, and throat specialist, but it was not developed and used until much later. According to Black, it is a challenging surgery to perform, but it can be very effective. The technique can give hope to patients whose tumors have deeply invaded their brains and for whom other surgical procedures may not be possible.

> " Brain specialists have long known that brain operations in which the skull is cut open carry serious potential risks for the patient.

In 2008 surgeons at New York-Presbyterian Hospital performed endoscopic surgery on a 50-year-old man. He had developed a tangerine-sized tumor on his pituitary gland. Though benign, the tumor was pressing on his optic nerve and spreading toward other parts of his brain. In a prior traditional operation involving removal of a section of the skull to reach the brain, a piece of the tumor was left in place and a second surgery was recommended. He decided to undergo the endoscopic procedure instead. Using long tubes tipped with cameras and miniaturized tools, the surgeons removed the tumor through the man's nasal passages. Within 2 weeks he was back on his feet and feeling better, and 1 year after the surgery he was completely recovered.

Radiation Therapy

After surgery has been performed and a brain tumor removed, patients often undergo radiation therapy. This technique uses high-energy rays (similar to X-rays) to destroy tumor tissue that remains in the brain, as well as to kill any remaining cancer cells. In cases where surgery is not possible, radiation therapy may be used in an attempt to shrink the tumor. The treatment may be given externally, using a large machine that beams radiation into a patient's head. Or radioactive material may be surgically placed in the tumor, which is known as implant radiation therapy.

There are, however, risks associated with radiation therapy, especially when it is directed toward the entire brain. Although it kills cancerous cells, it also destroys healthy cells in the process. As Black explains: "You can't really crank up the amount of whole brain radiation high enough to destroy the tumor without destroying a lot of healthy brain tissue; it's akin to swatting at fleas in a bearskin rug with a hatchet."[60] In young children radiation therapy can cause even worse problems than in adults, impairing their growth, learning, vision, and hearing. Because of the risks of radiation, some brain specialists are using a different type of treatment known as proton beam therapy.

> " Although the diagnosis of a brain tumor can be terrifying for anyone, people's chances of survival today are significantly better than they were in the past. "

The idea of proton beam therapy was first conceived in the 1950s. The first hospital-based treatment facility opened in California in 1990, but because the technology costs tens of millions of dollars, there are still only eight operating centers in the United States. Proton beam therapy uses small nuclear particles (known as protons) rather than electromagnetic radiation. Thus, it can precisely target abnormal cells without damaging adjacent healthy cells. According to the National Association for Proton Therapy, the treatment's precision ability allows a radiation oncologist to increase the dose to the tumor while reducing the dose to surrounding tissues, which is not possible with traditional types of radiation. The group writes "the overall affects lead to the potential for fewer harmful side effects, more direct impact on the tumor, and increased tumor control."[61]

One child who has benefited from proton beam therapy is 2-year-old Addison Keegan. Until February 2010 Addison was a healthy child who was developing normally, but then she became violently ill. Tests showed that a benign tumor was lodged in her brain stem. Neurosurgeons removed as much of it as they could, but radiation was still necessary to treat any residual tumor cells. She underwent proton beam therapy, during which high-dose radiation was delivered within 0.04 inches (1mm) of her tumor site. At the end of 30 treatments, Addison's MRI scans showed no trace of a tumor, and she suffered from no apparent side effects. "She's running around, just like she was," says her mother. "This is as good as I imagined it would be."[62]

Looking Toward the Future

Although the diagnosis of a brain tumor can be terrifying for anyone, people's chances of survival today are significantly better than they were in the past. Once MRI scans pinpoint the location of a tumor in someone's brain, advanced surgical techniques make it possible for many to be completely removed. Advanced technology such as proton beam therapy enables patients to undergo high-dose radiation treatments without damage to surrounding tissue. As scientists continue to develop sophisticated treatments, increasing numbers of brain tumor sufferers will undoubtedly be able to live longer than ever before. "Meanwhile," says Black, "the war goes on. We fight brain tumor battles on a daily basis, but one day we will win the war. That is something I *have* to believe."[63]

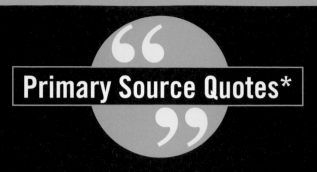

Primary Source Quotes*

How Successful Are Brain Tumor Treatments?

66 The promise of cures for difficult tumors is becoming a reality to more families than ever before. 99

—John R. Mangiardi, "Brain Tumors in Children," Brain and Neurosurgery Information Center, February 2010. www.brain-surgery.com.

Mangiardi is a New York neurosurgeon and the founder and author of the Brain and Neurosurgery Information Center Web site.

66 Targeted drug treatments focus on specific abnormalities present within cancer cells. By blocking these abnormalities, targeted drug treatments can cause cancer cells to die. 99

—Mayo Clinic, "Brain Tumor," May 15, 2010. www.mayoclinic.com.

The Mayo Clinic is a world-renowned medical facility headquartered in Rochester, Minnesota.

* Editor's Note: While the definition of a primary source can be narrowly or broadly defined, for the purposes of Compact Research, a primary source consists of: 1) results of original research presented by an organization or researcher; 2) eyewitness accounts of events, personal experience, or work experience; 3) first-person editorials offering pundits' opinions; 4) government officials presenting political plans and/or policies; 5) representatives of organizations presenting testimony or policy.

❝The location of a brain tumor will dictate whether or not surgery is an option. Some tumors are seated in places in the brain that are just too dangerous to operate on.❞

—Christopher Dolinsky, "Brain Cancer: The Basics," OncoLink, February 29, 2008. www.oncolink.org.

Dolinsky is a radiation oncologist at the Abramson Cancer Center of the University of Pennsylvania.

❝Radiation therapy fights cancer by damaging cancer cells with a powerful blast of energy.❞

—American Association for Cancer Research, "Brain Cancer," July 17, 2008. www.aacr.org.

The American Association for Cancer Research seeks to prevent and cure cancer through research, education, communication, and collaboration.

❝Chronic effects of prolonged radiation treatment tend to be more serious and range from impairment of intellectual capacity to complete incapacity.❞

—J. Stephen Huff, "Neoplasms, Brain," eMedicine, August 26, 2009. http://emedicine.medscape.com.

Huff is an emergency medicine and neurology professor at the University of Virginia's department of emergency medicine.

❝Today, more than half of all children diagnosed with a brain tumor will be cured of the disease.❞

—Children's Hospital Boston, "Brain Tumors," January 25, 2010. www.childrenshospital.org.

Children's Hospital Boston is one of the largest pediatric medical centers in the United States.

> **One problem with current therapies such as brain radiation and intensive chemotherapy is that they have major impacts on brain development in children. Consequently, brain tumor survivors often suffer from a number of life-long handicaps.**

—Gregory Plautz, "T Cell Immunotherapy for Malignant Brain Tumors," *Cancer Consult*, 2008. http://my.clevelandclinic.org.

Plautz is chair of the Department of Pediatric Hematology/Oncology at the Cleveland Clinic.

> **Although the prognosis of patients with malignant glioma has improved during the past decade, therapies currently under development are likely to improve the treatment of this devastating disease even more.**

—Maciej S. Lesniak, "Promising Developments in Treating Malignant Glioma," Dana Foundation, 2010. www.dana.org.

Lesniak is an associate professor of surgery and the director of neurosurgical oncology at the University of Chicago Medical Center's Brain Tumor Center.

> **Physicians believe that the number of patients diagnosed with brain metastases is on the rise because treatments for primary cancers are improving continually and patients are surviving with these diseases longer.**

—Memorial Sloan-Kettering Cancer Center, "Brain Tumors, Metastatic: Overview," April 28, 2009. www.mskcc.org.

The Memorial Sloan-Kettering Cancer Center is a world-renowned cancer facility that is headquartered in New York City.

How Successful Are
Brain Tumor Treatments?

- The U.S. Central Brain Tumor Registry states that on average, **35.1 percent** of people with malignant brain tumors survive for 2 years, **26.6 percent** for 5 years, and **22.2 percent** for 10 years.

- In 2010 the National Cancer Institute reported a **significant decrease** in the number of deaths from malignant brain tumors since 1975.

- The American Brain Tumor Association states that **more knowledge** about brain tumors has been gained in the past 10 years than in the past hundred years.

- The National Institutes of Health states that risks of radiation therapy for brain tumors include **stroke and dementia** (mental deterioration).

- Children's Hospital Boston states that more than **50 percent** of all children diagnosed with a brain tumor can be cured.

- According to neurosurgeon John R. Mangiardi, while radiation therapy works well at treating a brain tumor, the **brain damage** it causes can exceed the damage done by the tumor itself.

- According to the Mayo Clinic, alternative treatments such as **acupuncture, meditation, and hypnosis** have not been proved to cure brain tumors.

Improved Survival Rates

For many years, a malignant brain tumor diagnosis was considered a death sentence. Now, because medical science has resulted in numerous treatments, people with brain cancer are able to live longer than ever before. This was apparent in a 2010 report by the National Cancer Institute, which showed a steady rise in survival rates (with the greatest among males) from 1975 to 2006.

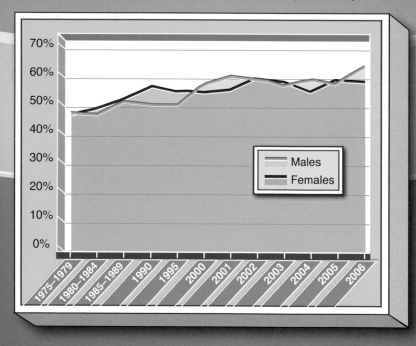

**One-Year Survival Rates
1975–2006, Males and Females (Percent)**

Source: National Cancer Institute, *SEER Cancer Statistics Review, 1975–2007*, June 30, 2010. http://seer.cancer.gov.

- The American Cancer Society states that children with malignant brain tumors had a **72 percent** survival rate between 1995 and 2006.

- According to the American Cancer Society, the five-year survival rate for people with malignant brain tumors who are over 75 is still only about **5 percent**.

Health Insurance a Challenge for Brain Tumor Patients

A number of treatments can help people who suffer from brain tumors and markedly improve their chances of survival. For various reasons, however, brain tumor patients are not always able to take advantage of available treatments. In a 2008 poll by the American Brain Tumor Association, participants shared the challenges they face in efforts to obtain treatment for themselves or for family members.

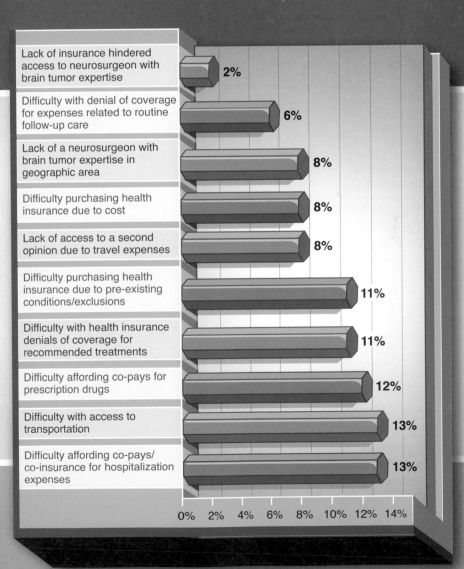

Challenge	Percentage
Lack of insurance hindered access to neurosurgeon with brain tumor expertise	2%
Difficulty with denial of coverage for expenses related to routine follow-up care	6%
Lack of a neurosurgeon with brain tumor expertise in geographic area	8%
Difficulty purchasing health insurance due to cost	8%
Lack of access to a second opinion due to travel expenses	8%
Difficulty purchasing health insurance due to pre-existing conditions/exclusions	11%
Difficulty with health insurance denials of coverage for recommended treatments	11%
Difficulty affording co-pays for prescription drugs	12%
Difficulty with access to transportation	13%
Difficulty affording co-pays/co-insurance for hospitalization expenses	13%

Source: American Brain Tumor Association, "Survey: Top Challenges to Optimal Care," Fall 2008. www.abta.org.

When Surgery Is Not Possible

Neurosurgery is highly sophisticated today, and can help people with brain tumors live long, healthy lives, often free from symptoms. But not everyone who suffers from brain tumors is able to undergo surgery.

When Brain Surgery Might Not Be Recommended

Location of the tumor	If the tumor is deep in the brain, it may not be accessible without the risk of severe damage (such as tumors located in the brain stem and thalamus); tumors may also present a problem if they are located near sensitive areas that control language, movement, vision, or other critical functions.
Diagnosis and size of tumor	If the tumor is benign, does not cause pressure on the brain (due to small size), or cause problems with sensitive areas, avoiding or post-poning surgery might be the patient's best option.
Number of tumors	The presence of multiple tumors creates additional challenges to safe removal.
Border (or edges) of a tumor	If a tumor's edges are poorly defined, it may be mixed in with normal brain tissue and be difficult to remove completely.
Patient's general health	A patient's heart, lungs, liver, and overall general health must be strong enough to endure surgery.
Patient's neurological status	Existing symptoms of pressure within the brain, or signs of nerve damage, need to be evaluated before surgery is attempted.
Previous surgery	If a patient has had recent surgery, it is usually necessary for him/her to recover completely before going through another operation.
Other options	The physician may determine that an alternative treatment would provide equal or better results at a comparable or lower risk.

Source: American Brain Tumor Association, *Focusing on Treatment: Surgery*, 2004. www.abta.org.

- Neurosurgeon John R. Mangiardi states that in order for treatment to cure a brain tumor, it **must treat the entire brain**, reach every tumor cell, kill all cell types within the tumor, and spare the remaining normal brain.

- Children's Hospital Boston states that benign tumors remain well **encapsulated** in the brain and complete surgical removal is usually sufficient treatment.

- Following brain tumor surgery, **extensive rehabilitation** may be necessary to help a patient recover lost motor skills, as well as speech, vision, and thinking skills.

Key People and Advocacy Groups

American Brain Tumor Association: An organization that funds research with a focus on brain tumor diagnosis, treatment, and care, with the ultimate goal of finding a cure.

American Cancer Society: An organization that seeks to eliminate cancer as a major health problem by preventing it and saving lives through research, education, advocacy, and service.

Keith Black: Considered one of the top neurosurgeons in the world, Black is the director of the Maxine Dunitz Neurosurgical Institute at Cedars-Sinai Medical Center in Los Angeles.

Brain Tumor Foundation for Children: An organization that provides assistance and support for families of children with brain and spinal cord tumors, funds research, and works to raise public awareness of the disease.

Children's Brain Tumor Foundation: A group that seeks to improve the quality of life and long-term outlook for children with brain and spinal cord tumors through research, support, education, and advocacy.

Harvey Cushing: Now called the father of neurological surgery, Cushing was the first to develop basic techniques and instruments for operating on the brain in the earth twentieth century.

Vini Khurana: A prominent neurosurgeon who announced in 2008 that cell phones have the potential to kill more people than smoking or asbestos.

National Brain Tumor Society: An organization that seeks to find a cure and improve the quality of life for those affected by brain tumors through research and support services.

National Cancer Institute: An agency of the National Institutes of Health and the U.S. government's principal federal agency for cancer research and training.

Pediatric Brain Tumor Foundation: An organization that exists to increase public awareness of the severity and prevalence of childhood brain tumors, support medical research, and provide support for children who suffer from brain tumors and their families.

Wilder Penfield: A neurosurgeon who, along with anesthesiologist André Pasquet, developed the awake craniotomy, a type of brain surgery that is performed while the patient is awake and able to communicate with doctors.

Karl Thiersch: A German surgeon who showed that cancers metastasize through the spread of malignant cells and not through some unidentified fluid, as was previously theorized.

Chronology

1761
Italian pathologist Giovanni Battista Morgagni publishes a textbook in which he describes cancers based on the findings compiled from 700 autopsies. This lays the foundation for scientific oncology, the study of cancer.

1896
German physicist Wilhelm Roentgen presents a lecture in which he describes his discovery of X-rays. Within months X-ray diagnostic systems are being designed, and within three years radiation is being used to treat cancer.

1838
Johannes Müller observes cancerous tissue under a microscope and postulates that cancer cells arise from a mass of cell-like fluids known as a blastema. This theory, known as the blastema theory of cancer, is later proved to be incorrect.

1750   **1825**   **1900**

1779
The first cancer hospital in France is forced to move away from the city of Reims because of the erroneous belief that cancer is contagious.

1839
French gynecologist Joseph Récamier describes the invasion of the bloodstream by cancer cells, coining the word *metastasis* to describe the spread of cancer.

1865
German surgeon Karl Thiersch shows that cancers metastasize through the spread of malignant cells, rather than through unidentified fluid as was previously believed.

1858
German pathologist Rudolf Virchow, a pupil of Johannes Müller, disproves the blastema theory and confirms that cancer cells arise from preexisting cells.

1968
Swedish neurosurgeon Lars Leksell and his colleague, Börje Larsson, introduce the gamma knife, which treats brain tumors with high-energy electromagnetic beams that target a small area without harming healthy brain tissue.

2010
Robert Wood Johnson University Hospital in New Brunswick, New Jersey, becomes the first hospital in the United States to perform laser-assisted surgery (which destroys a tumor with heat) on a rare tumor that grows from the cells that line the brain's ventricles.

1972
American scientist Raymond Damadian receives a patent for his invention, the magnetic resonance scanner, which eventually becomes the premier diagnostic imaging technique.

1995
The National Cancer Institute reports that of the 2,275 cancer deaths of children and youth aged 19 and under, nearly one-fourth are due to malignant tumors of the brain and central nervous system.

1960

1985

2010

1971
British engineer Godfrey Hounsfield creates an instrument that combines X-rays with computer technology and calls it computerized tomography, which becomes invaluable for scanning the brain for tumors and also for guiding biopsy needles into tumors.

1978
Baltimore Brain Tumor Research Center director Michael Walker and his colleagues prove that radiation treatment (X-ray therapy) significantly prolongs life for patients with malignant astrocytomas, tumors that arise from star-shaped brain cells called astrocytes.

2005
Researchers at the University of California–Los Angeles identify genetic characteristics that make some brain tumors 51 times more likely to respond to a specific class of drugs, a finding that could help avoid therapies that might not benefit some patients.

1977
In performing the first scan of the entire human body, Raymond Damadian proves that magnetic resonance technology is superior to X-rays for viewing the body's vital organs.

2009
Edward Kennedy, one of the longest-serving members of the U.S. Senate, dies 15 months after being diagnosed with a malignant brain tumor.

Related Organizations

American Brain Tumor Association

2720 River Rd.
Des Plaines, IL 60018
phone: (847) 827-9910 • fax: (847) 827-9918
e-mail: info@abta.org • Web site: www.abta.org

The American Brain Tumor Association funds research that is focused on brain tumor diagnosis, treatment, and care, with the ultimate goal of finding a cure. Its Web site features numerous articles about brain tumors, a comprehensive booklet titled *A Primer of Brain Tumors*, a *Facts & Statistics 2010* document, and information about research.

American Cancer Society

250 Williams St. NW, Suite 6000
Atlanta, GA 30303
phone: (404) 320-3333; toll-free: (800) 227-2345
Web site: www.cancer.org

The American Cancer Society seeks to eliminate cancer as a major health problem by saving lives through research, education, advocacy, and service. Its Web site offers a comprehensive *Cancer Facts & Figures 2010* booklet, news releases, Dr. Len's Cancer Blog, and a search engine that produces hundreds of articles about brain tumors and cancer.

Brain Science Foundation

148 Linden St., Suite 303
Wellesley, MA 02482
phone: (781) 239-2903; toll-free: (866) 492-2466 • fax: (781) 239-2907
e-mail: info@brainsciencefoundation.org
Web site: www.brainsciencefoundation.org

The Brain Science Foundation seeks to increase awareness of primary brain tumors and to make brain tumor research a priority. Its Web site offers information about types of brain tumors as well as symptoms, diagnosis, and treatment options. Also on the site is an assortment of fact sheets, news articles, and videos of patient stories.

Brain Tumor Foundation for Children

6065 Roswell Rd., Suite 505
Atlanta, GA 30328
phone: (404) 252-4107 • fax: (404) 252-4108
e-mail: info@braintumorkids.org • Web site: www.braintumorkids.org

The Brain Tumor Foundation for Children provides assistance and support for families of children with brain and spinal cord tumors, funds research, and works to raise public awareness of the disease. Its Web site features an Information and Resources section, a link to the Butterfly Blog, and archived news articles.

Childhood Brain Tumor Foundation

20312 Watkins Meadow Dr.
Germantown, MD 20876
phone: (301) 515-2900; toll free: (877) 217-4166
e-mail: cbtf@childhoodbraintumor.org
Web site: www.childhoodbraintumor.org

The Childhood Brain Tumor Foundation raises funds for scientific research and seeks to heighten public awareness and to improve the prognosis and quality of life for those affected by brain tumors. Its Web site offers an online newsletter, webcasts, and a collection of articles and stories about brain tumors.

Children's Brain Tumor Foundation

274 Madison Ave., Suite 1004
New York, NY 10016
phone: (212) 448-9494; toll free: (866) 228-4673
e-mail: info@cbtf.org • Web site: www.cbtf.org

The Children's Brain Tumor Foundation seeks to improve the quality of life and long-term outlook for children with brain and spinal cord tumors through research, support, education, and advocacy. Its Web site offers a wide array of information about brain tumors including a Facts and Glossary section, research news, a link to a blog, and an online discussion forum.

I'm Too Young for This! Cancer Foundation

40 Worth St., Suite 808
New York, NY 10013
phone: toll-free: (877) 735-4673 • fax: (877) 794-6902
e-mail: into@i2y.com • Web site: http://i2y.com

The I'm Too Young for This! Cancer Foundation works exclusively on behalf of cancer survivors under the age of 40. Its Web site is tailored toward young people and features news articles, the Stupid Cancer Blog, newsletters, essays, and a Support Channels section that links to forums, chat rooms, and other resources.

National Cancer Institute

NCI Office of Communications and Education
Public Inquiries Office
6116 Executive Blvd., Suite 300
Bethesda, MD 20892-8322
phone: (301) 496-1038; toll-free: (800) 422-6237
e-mail: cancergovstaff@mail.nih.gov • Web site: www.cancer.gov

An agency of the National Institutes of Health, the National Cancer Institute is the U.S. government's principal federal agency for cancer research and training. A wealth of information is available on its Web site, including cancer statistics, fact sheets, news releases, clinical trial results, and a link to the separate Brain Tumor site.

National Institute for Neurological Disorders and Stroke (NINDS)

PO Box 5801
Bethesda, MD 20824
phone: (301) 496-5751; toll-free: (800) 352-9424 • fax: (301) 402-2060
Web site: www.ninds.nih.gov

An agency of the National Institutes of Health, the NINDS seeks to reduce the burden of neurological disease through research and education. Its Brain and Spinal Tumors Information Page produces a number of informative publications, including "Brain and Spinal Tumors: Hope Through Research."

North American Brain Tumor Coalition

Turner & Goss LLP
2446 Thirty-ninth St. NW
Washington, DC 20007
phone: (202) 508-4670 • fax: (202) 508-4650
e-mail: info@nabraintumor.org • Web site: www.nabraintumor.org

The North American Brain Tumor Coalition works to advance the interests of people with brain tumors through coordinated and cooperative public policy efforts. Its Web site features facts about brain tumors, news releases, and archived articles that cover research, advocacy, and general news.

Pediatric Brain Tumor Foundation

302 Ridgefield Ct.
Asheville, NC 28806
phone: (828) 665-6891; toll-free: (800) 253-6530 • fax: (828) 665-6894
e-mail: pbtfus@pbtfus.org • Web site: www.pbtfus.org

The Pediatric Brain Tumor Foundation exists to increase public awareness of the severity and prevalence of childhood brain tumors, support medical research, and provide support for children who suffer from brain tumors and their families. Its Web site features *The Caring Hand* newsletter, personal stories of survival, news articles, and informative brain tumor booklets.

For Further Research

Books

Keith Black, *Brain Surgeon*. New York: Wellness Central-Hatchett Book Group, 2009.

Ayis A. Caperonis, *Stepping over Myself: Finding My Way and My Life After a Brain Tumor*. Bloomington, IN: AuthorHouse, 2009.

Brooke Desserich and Keith Desserich, *Notes Left Behind*. New York: William Morrow, 2009.

Les Duncan, *Brain Storms: Surviving Catastrophic Illness*. Mustang, OK: Tate, 2008.

Katrina Firlik, *Another Day in the Frontal Lobe: A Brain Surgeon Exposes Life on the Inside*. New York: Random House, 2007.

Liz Holzemer, *Curveball: When Life Throws You a Brain Tumor*. Denver, CO: Ghost Road, 2007.

Virginia Stark-Vance and M.L. Dubay, *100 Questions & Answers About Brain Tumors*. Sudbury, MA: Jones and Bartlett, 2011.

Tim B. Ward, *Surviving and Thriving: A Brain Tumor Survivor's Story*. Parker, CO: Outskirts, 2010.

Periodicals

Coco Ballantyne, "Fetal Stem Cells Cause Tumor in a Teenage Boy," *Scientific American*, February 19, 2009.

Christopher Ketcham, "Warning: Your Cell Phone May Be Hazardous to Your Health," *GQ*, February 2010.

Rachel Mehlhaff, "Girl Fights Against Rare Brain Tumor," *Denton (TX) Record-Chronicle*, May 31, 2010.

Brian Newsome, "'I've Never Seen Anything Like It,' Doctor Says of Newborn's Brain Surgery," *Colorado Springs Gazette*, December 15, 2008.

New York Times, "Brain Tumor—Primary—Adults," October 14, 2009. http://health.nytimes.com.

Tiffany O'Callaghan, "A Way to Keep Brain Tumors from Coming Back?" *Time*, February 23, 2010.

Tara Parker-Pope, "Experts Revive Debate over Cellphones and Cancer," *New York Times*, June 3, 2008.

Kevin Poulsen, "'Known Software Bug' Disrupts Brain Tumor Zapping," *Wired*, October 16, 2009.

Steven Reinberg, "Brain Tumor Drug May Help Spur Cancer's Return," *U.S. News & World Report*, March 5, 2009.

Sabin Russell, "No Cure for Malignant Glioma Like Kennedy Has," *San Francisco Chronicle*, May 21, 2008.

Victoria Stern, "Does Herpes Cause Brain Cancer?" *Scientific American*, August 2008.

Tara Subkoff, "I Survived a Brain Tumor," *Harper's Bazaar*, May 2010.

Internet Sources

American Brain Tumor Association, "A Primer of Brain Tumors," January 2009. www.abta.org/index.cfm?contentid=170&Primer-Basic tumorinformation.

John R. Mangiardi, "A, B, C's of Brain Tumors," Brain and Neurosurgery Information Center, February 2010. www.brain-surgery.com/primer.html.

National Cancer Institute, *What You Need to Know About Brain Tumors*, May 2009. www.cancer.gov/cancertopics/wyntk/brain.pdf.

National Institute of Health, "Brain Tumors," National Library of Medicine, Medline Plus, April 30, 2008. www.nlm.nih.gov/medlineplus/tutorials/braincancer/oc119103.pdf.

Source Notes

Overview

1. Tara Subkoff, "I Survived a Brain Tumor," *Harper's Bazaar*, May 2010, p. 155.
2. Subkoff, "I Survived a Brain Tumor," p. 157.
3. Keith Black, *Brain Surgeon*. New York: Wellness Central-Hatchett Book Group, 2009, p. xi.
4. Daniel Silverman and Idelle Davidson, *Your Brain After Chemo*. Cambridge, MA: DeCapo, 2009, p. 92.
5. Bruce Goldman, "Gray Matters: Unsung Brain Cells Determine Function of Neurons, Researchers Discover," news release, Stanford Medical School, September 21, 2009. http://med.stanford.edu.
6. University of Utah Genetic Science Learning Center, "The Other Brain Cells," 2010. http://learn.genetics.utah.edu.
7. American Cancer Society, *Testing Biology and Cytology Specimens for Cancer*, March 24, 2010. www.cancer.org.
8. Don M. Long, "Gliomas: The Latest Research," Dana Foundation, May 29, 2008. www.dana.org.
9. American Brain Tumor Association, "Facts & Statistics," 2010. www.abta.org.
10. Peter M. Black, "Tumors of Childhood—The Dana Guide," Dana Foundation, *The Dana Guide to Brain Health*, March 2007. www.dana.org.
11. Children's Hospital Boston, "Brain Tumors," January 25, 2010. www.childrenshospital.org.
12. Quoted in MSNBC, "Kennedy's Tumor Was Aggressive and Deadly," August 26, 2009. www.msnbc.msn.com.
13. National Brain Tumor Society, "Brain Tumor FAQ," 2010. www.braintumor.org.
14. Black, *Brain Surgeon*, p. 4.
15. Lisa M. DeAngelis, "Brain Tumors—The Dana Guide," Dana Foundation, *The Dana Guide to Brain Health*, June 2009. www.dana.org.

What Are Brain Tumors?

16. Quoted in Jan Klooster, "Fundraiser to Help Mesick Teen with Brain Tumor," *Cadillac News*, August 20, 2010. www.cadillacnews.com.
17. Caitlin DeVoll, e-mail interview with author, September 17, 2010.
18. Donald Ingber, "Ingber's Egg Analogy," Children's Hospital Boston, 2006. www.childrenshospital.org.
19. Ingber, "Ingber's Egg Analogy."
20. Ingber, "Ingber's Egg Analogy."
21. University of California–San Francisco Medical Center, "Brain Tumor," July 31, 2007. www.ucsfhealth.org.
22. Black, *Brain Surgeon*, p. 52.
23. Memorial Sloan-Kettering Cancer Center, "Brain Tumors, Metastatic: Overview," April 28, 2009. www.mskcc.org.
24. Christopher Dolinsky, "Brain Cancer: The Basics," OncoLink, February 29, 2008. www.oncolink.org.
25. Olivia Briggs, "The Truth About 'Benign' Brain Tumors," Associated Content, May 27, 2009. www.associated-content.com.
26. Quoted in Mike Celizic, "Baby OK After Surgeons Remove Foot from His Brain," *Today*, NBC News, January 13, 2009. http://today.msnbc.msn.com.
27. Quoted in Denver Channel, "Colorado Doctor Finds Foot in Newborn's

Brain," December 17, 2008. www.thedenverchannel.com.

What Causes Brain Tumors?

28. John R. Mangiardi, "A, B, C's of Brain Tumors," Brain and Neurosurgery Information Center, February 2010. www.brain-surgery.com.

29. National Cancer Institute, *What You Need to Know About Brain Tumors*, May 2009. www.cancer.gov.

30. Dolinsky, "Brain Cancer."

31. American Cancer Society, "Childhood Cancer: Late Effects of Cancer Treatments," 2009. www.cancer.org.

32. Dave Embrey, "Mom Just Diagnosed with Tumor in Her Brain," National Brain Tumor Society, April 20, 2010. http://my.braintumorcommunity.org.

33. Dolinsky, "Brain Cancer."

34. Quoted in Greg Allen, "Cancer Cluster in Florida Worries Parents," NPR, April 5, 2010. www.npr.org.

35. Quoted in University of Oxford, "Study Reveals How Cancers Spread to the Brain," June 10, 2009. www.ox.ac.uk.

36. Quoted in Asher Moses, "Brain Cancer Fears over Heavy Mobile Phone Use," *Sydney Morning Herald*, March 31, 2008. www.smh.com.au.

37. Quoted in International Agency for Research on Cancer, "Interphone Study Reports on Mobile Phone Use and Brain Cancer Risk," press release, May 17, 2010. www.iarc.fr.

38. Quoted in Janet Raloff, "Interphone Study Finds Hints of Brain Cancer Risk in Heavy Cell-Phone Users," Science News, May 17, 2010. www.sciencenews.org.

What Are the Risks of Brain Tumors?

39. Martin L. Lazar, "Chordoma," Neurosurgical Consultants, May 9, 2010. www.neurosurgerydallas.com.

40. Black, *Brain Surgeon*, p. 44.

41. Black, *Brain Surgeon*, p. 45.

42. Black, *Brain Surgeon*, p. 44.

43. Black, *Brain Surgeon*, p. 212.

44. Mangiardi, "A, B, C's of Brain Tumors."

45. Children's Brain Tumor Foundation, "Educational Late Effects," November 11, 2009. www.cbtf.org.

46. American Brain Tumor Association, "Seizures," 2010. www.abta.org.

47. Quoted in Katherine Lee, "Understanding the Effects of Seizures on Children," Everyday Health, March 5, 2009. www.everydayhealth.com.

48. Mayo Clinic, "Absence Seizure (Petit Mal Seizure)," June 23, 2009. www.mayoclinic.com.

49. Katie Rozenas, "My Battle with Cushing's Disease," Children's Hospital Boston, *Dream Online*, Winter 2009. www.childrenshospital.org.

50. Rozenas, "My Battle with Cushing's Disease."

51. Rozenas, "My Battle with Cushing's Disease."

52. Quoted in Matthew Cyr, "One in 10 Million," *Dream*, Winter 2009. http://web1.tch.harvard.edu.

How Successful Are Brain Tumor Treatments?

53. Quoted in Michael Carvell, "Two Brain Surgeries Can't Stop Kell High Star," *Atlanta Journal-Constitution*, October 13, 2009. www.ajc.com.

54. Quoted in James Carlton, "Georgia Star Paul Amend Refused to Let Brain Tumor Break His Spirit," *Sports Illustrated*, February 26, 2010. http://sportsillustrated.cnn.com.

55. Long, "Gliomas: The Latest Research."

56. Denni Proctor, "A Gift for Katie Proctor & Friends," Pediatric Brain Tumor Foundation First Giving, Summer 2010. www.firstgiving.com.

57. Black, *Brain Surgeon*, pp. 52–53.
58. Black, *Brain Surgeon*, p. 206.
59. Quoted in New York Presbyterian, "Surgeons Remove Giant Brain Tumor with New, Minimally Invasive Technique," news release, March 1, 2009. http://nyp.org.
60. Black, *Brain Surgeon*, p. 61.
61. National Association for Proton Therapy, "How It Works," 2010. www.proton-therapy.org.
62. Quoted in Sanjay Gupta, "Hope for Children with Brain Tumors," CBS News, May 26, 2010. www.onlinecancerguide.com.
63. Black, *Brain Surgeon*, p. 221.

List of Illustrations

Index

Note: Page numbers in boldface indicate illustrations.

About the Author

Peggy J. Parks holds a bachelor of science degree from Aquinas College in Grand Rapids, Michigan, where she graduated magna cum laude. An author who has written nearly 100 educational books for children and young adults, Parks lives in Muskegon, Michigan, a town that she says inspires her writing because of its location on the shores of Lake Michigan.